SUCCESSFUL LIVING
WITH CHRONIC ILLNESS

SUCCESSFUL
LIVING
WITH CHRONIC ILLNESS

Kathleen S. Lewis

AVERY PUBLISHING GROUP INC.
Wayne, New Jersey

The therapeutic procedures in this book are based on the training, personal experiences, and research of the author. Because each person and situation is unique, the author and publisher urge the reader to check with a qualified health professional before using any procedure where there is any question as to its appropriateness.

The publisher does not advocate the use of any particular program, but believes the information presented in this book should be available to the public.

Because there is always some risk involved, the author and publisher are not responsible for any adverse effects or consequences resulting from the use of any of the suggestions or procedures in this book. Please do not use the book if you are unwilling to assume the risk. Feel free to consult a physician or other qualified health professional. It is a sign of wisdom, not cowardice, to seek a second or third opinion.

Cover design by Martin Hochberg and Rudy Shur
In-house editor Jacqueline Balla
Layout designed by Diana Puglisi
Typesetting by ACS Graphic Services, Fresh Meadows, NY

Library of Congress Cataloging in Publication Data
Lewis, Kathleen S., 1944-
  Successful living with chronic illness.

  Articles from the author's Let's celebrate life
column in Horizons newsletter, 1981-1984.
  Bibliography: p.
  Includes index.
  1. Chronically ill--Psychology--Addresses, essays,
lectures. 2. Chronically ill--Care and treatment--
Addresses, essays, lectures. 3. Adjustment
(Psychology)--Addresses, essays, lectures.
I. Title.
R726.5.L49 1985   362.1   85-13494
ISBN 0-89529-296-3 (pbk.)

Printed in the United States of America

10 9 8 7 6 5 4 3 2 1

Contents

Dedication

I would like to dedicate this book to Jim, my husband / lover / advisor / comforter / confidant / partner / "go-fer" / and friend, without whom I would never have been able to "make it through the rain and keep my own perspective, make it through the rain and keep my point of view, make it through the rain and find myself respected by others who were rained on, too, and made it through."*

---

*From "I Made it Through the Rain," by Gerard Kenny, Drey Shepperd, Barry Manilow, Jack Feldman, and Bruce Sussman. Copyright © 1979 & 1980 by D & J Arlon Enterprises Ltd. Published in the U.S.A. by Unichappell Music, Inc. International Copyright Secured. ALL RIGHTS RESERVED. Used by permission.

Acknowledgements

I would like to acknowledge Jeanette M. Walters, my typist / editor / friend and President of The Lupus Foundation, Greater Atlanta Chapter who diligently, patiently, and faithfully picked through my awful typing, hen-scratching, and arrows; Penny Willibey, who was always there with her typing skills and friendship when I was in a pinch; Bob G. Lanier, M.D., my primary physician / co-worker / friend, who was among the few who encouraged my feeble writing efforts; Don Cabaniss, Ph.D., Acting Director of Pastoral Care Program at Georgia Baptist Medical Center, Atlanta, Georgia, who is my teacher / counselor / chaplain / mentor / friend; the many patients who shared their journeys with me; Jamie and Keith Lewis, my two teenage sons, who see me at my best and my worst; many nurturing, caring, loving, and faithful people I have had the privilege of calling my friends (you know who you are); and The Lupus Foundation of America, Inc., Greater Atlanta Chapter, for allowing my articles to find their first audience in *Horizons*, our monthly newsletter.

Foreword

About two years ago I received an unsolicited manuscript concerning living with chronic illness, which its author asked me, in my role as editor-in-chief of *Postgraduate Medicine*, to consider for publication. The subject is an important one for the doctors our journal serves—family physicians, general internists, and other primary care physicians—but, frankly, not a very exciting one. The submitted manuscript did little to spark my interest. It was dull and pedantic, filled with psychobabble.

I returned the essay to the author with a candid opinion, pointing out the rather stilted language and stating my belief that our readers simply would not read this. Having rejected the article, I quickly put it out of my mind. Therefore, I was somewhat surprised to receive a revised manuscript a few weeks later.

"Revised" is an inadequate term, however, to describe this new manuscript, which bore little or no resemblance to the earlier version. I was now reading a compassionate, personal, and moving account of living with a chronic illness—the ups and downs, the sadness and grief, the changes in life-style and in personal relationships that occur when one is so afflicted. I promptly accepted this article, and it was published under the title, "Living with Chronic Illness: Dying is the Easy Part," in our September 1983 issue. It has been reproduced beginning on page 45 of this volume.

This experience constituted my introduction to Kathleen S. Lewis. Subsequently, through continuing correspondence, I have come to know her as an unusually gifted person, a person with special perceptions and inspired insights that she shares with us here. Her intelligence, her strength of will, and her intense religious faith are all evident throughout.

Ms. Lewis' work deserves to be read by physicians, who will be immensely helped in their understanding of what their chronically ill patients are going through. It should be read by friends and relatives of such patients, people who are so essential in constituting the support group for the sick person. These people will find out how important their roles are and learn much about how they may best fulfill them.

Most importantly, of course, the book should be read by every patient suffering from a chronic disease. It is a rich compendium of philosophical advice that concerns dealing with and ultimately accepting one's infirmity, as well as a group of helpful pragmatic hints about dealing with specific situations, such as visiting one's doctor. We should be grateful to Ms. Lewis for shedding new light on this shadowed area.

Robert B. Howard, MD

Introduction

When I started writing *Successful Living with Chronic Illness* in March, 1981, to be published as a column, "Let's Celebrate Life," in the Lupus Foundation of America, Inc., Greater Atlanta Chapter's newsletter, *Horizons*, I never dreamed that it would run as long as it has, be published as a collection in book form, or touch the lives of others, shedding some light on their way as it has!

Each article began with sweat, tears, and work. Grains of discomfort rubbing in my soul evolved into pearls of understanding —a lesson was learned, a truth discerned, or an insight gained. A part of me—my struggles, my defeats, and my victories—is laid out on each page in the hope that it will help at least one other person in his journey with chronic illness, whether he be a professional, family member, friend, or patient.

I have been privileged to see chronic illness from many different perspectives. I was prepared to write these articles in a school of nursing, while working as a nurse and nurse educator in many varied fields, as a citizen of the world of health. I then became a student with chronic illness in the school of the living, joining the ranks of the officially disabled. I discovered principles and lessons of successful living with chronic illness to be verified and reinforced later on by textbooks and teachers. I have completed an introductory course in pastoral care. I am struggling to become a free-lance writer, and working at a snail's pace on a masters degree in rehabilitation counseling.

I have learned more as a patient–professional in the school of learning to live with chronic illness than I ever did as just a professional. Lessons that were merely on paper have become a living reality, defined by personal experience never to be forgotten. It's a school I'll never graduate from, nor carry any degrees or titles except that of a "fellow struggler."

In this school I have come to be more in touch with my humanity and weaknesses, as well as unknown strengths and talents. I have learned that: the emotional response to chronic illness can be more crippling than the illness itself; being disabled doesn't mean you fall off the end of the earth never to return to the land of the living, for there are abilities within a disability; you can be rehabilitated within a disability without returning to substantial gainful employment; life does go on and can be full even though a former lifestyle is erased almost completely by chronic illness; even if the miracle of healing doesn't occur, that "wholing" within the context of chronic illness can be an even greater miracle; relationships are precious, for these contain the wealth of life; you need to learn to *live* to the edge of your cliff without going over by listening to what your body has to say; success in living with ongoing illness means learning to *live* joyfully where you are in the midst of illness and to celebrate *all* of life, the good and the bad; success in living can't be found in worldly standards and accomplishments but only in assuming responsibility for yourself and being faithful to yourself and to your Lord, and being persistent in your striving to give your best effort moment by moment no matter what the circumstances.

Successful Living with Chronic Illness is no longer mine and has become above and beyond anything I could have created or written. It has taken on its own being and has a life of its own in the lives of those who read it and reap benefits from it. Words confined to paper have become a part of the lives of others and have come to life. My life is but a speck in the dust of time, yet *Successful Living with Chronic Illness* will live on.

I hope that I can continue to learn and grow in the school of chronic illness and continue sharing more pearls with others in the same school, as they share theirs with me. I hope and pray that these pages will enrich the lives of others as their lives have enriched mine, and that we may strive to be successful in living with chronic illness by learning to embrace and celebrate *all* of life together as a precious gift, no matter what the circumstances.

There can be victory in defeat,
gain in loss,
living in dying,
wholeness in brokenness,
giving in receiving,
receiving in giving,
success in failure,
strength in weakness,
peace in turmoil,
joy in sorrow,
growth in pain, and
mental health in the midst of physical illness!
The crap and the tears can be transformed into fertilizer and rain for the soul to grow.

PART I

Relating to Others

1

The "$64,000 Question"

"How are you?" can perhaps become the most difficult question a chronically ill person needs to learn to answer. A question, once asked and answered in passing with no thought, may become a delicate moment where many factors must be carefully weighed.

Anger, bitterness, and a sense of isolation may result from such encounters until the person comes to better understand the transactions that take place in those brief exchanges. It may take some time for you to become comfortable with yourself and others in these moments.

You may be tempted to genuinely share how things really are, only to be challenged with: ". . . But you *look so good!*" Instead of being received as a compliment with appropriate thanks returned, it can come across as a put-down or denial of the situation just shared. An additional difficulty is added to an already sticky situation. There may be a loss of words in knowing how to respond for both parties.

Let's take a look at some of the things that may be going on with the people in this setting. You may desperately want to be understood and your difficult situation appreciated. Deciding "how you are" may be a task that could only be undertaken by a sophisticated computer, since illness may affect many varied bodily functions. "How you are" at some point in time may really only be determined in retrospect.

Wounds from past encounters may have taught you to clam up and not expose any real parts of yourself, cutting off any chances of communication. You may go to great lengths to hide your illness, due to embarrassment or self-consciousness. Also, saying you're sick all the time gets awkward, repetitious, and hard for others to hear.

The person asking the question may not really want to know "how you are." They may just be phrasing a socially accepted inquiry and not really expect an answer. It may be a ploy to solicit an inquiry as to their own well-being.

People are generally frightened by illness or someone who is different. Difficulties of others may be a threatening reminder of their own vulnerability. Denying their own human frailties, they must also deny them in others. People tend to avoid or run from those who ask them to understand more than they can understand, making them uncomfortable.

Those in the world of chronic illness may actually speak a different language from those in the world of health. They may use the same words but attach entirely different meanings to them. "Illness" in the world of the healthy may conjure up thoughts of acute problems with a duration of a few days, weeks, or months with medications that give quick answers or easy solutions.

Illness for the incurably, chronically ill means a lifetime of days upon days filled with ongoing, fluctuating health problems that have no easy solutions or quick answers. For the healthy, there may be the concept that you either get well or you die. There's no real understanding of getting sick, staying sick, and never really feeling well.

Our culture tends to see value and rewards only in quick solutions with visible results. Unsolvable problems, such as chronic illness, may be viewed as failures rather than challenges. Surely there's a pill for every ache and a cure for every problem?!

It isn't until those in the world of health walk through and experience days and months with those in the world of illness that the healthy can even begin to get beyond a surface understanding. Even at that, the understanding will be limited. You must realize the dimensions of the chasm to begin to calculate the problems.

Even in health, there are only a precious few with whom you can share the depths of your soul and circumstances. Identifying these special support persons and using them effectively is especially crucial for the chronically ill. Knowing there are those who care, though they may be few in number, can lessen the sting of the reality of what may seem to be indifference or avoidance from the majority of people encountered.

Understanding the dynamics of these encounters may help the long-term hurt begin to heal, but that still leaves you in the quandary of knowing how to respond in the situation. As a general rule, a response of: "I'm okay . . . fair . . . making it" may suffice and then allow the inquirer to seek his own level of interest.

You can allude to the presence of coping with difficulties by replies such as: "I've been better and I've been worse," "fair, some good and some bad," "I'm grinning and shuffling," "I'm hanging in there," "I'm keeping my head above water."

A direct way to probe the situation with someone you know well is to jokingly ask, "Do you want a lie, or do you want the truth?!" Learning ways to use humor puts you and others at ease and puts your circumstances in perspective.

Some comebacks to, "But you *look so good!*" might be: "Well, I really work at it," "War paint can work wonders," "Thank goodness, all that beauty rest does some good," "You look pretty good yourself," or, just a simple "Thank you!" Realizing you'll never get anywhere trying to prove that looks don't give the whole story may save some futile attempts to do so. When you try to prove something to someone, you give them control over you.

Continuing to look good during chronic illness, as many people do, can be a mixed blessing. The way you look is something highly valued in our society. You may be torn between covering the illness effects with make-up and looking the best that you can, or letting it all "hang out" so all or any of your illness effects will be visible, unquestionable, and undeniable to everyone you meet. The old saying, "If you look good, you'll feel good," presents unique problems here. You may look great but really feel lousy! The general assumption made by others may be that if you look great, then you must feel great.

The phrase that may unconsciously be left out is that looking great may correspond to feeling good or bad about yourself. How you feel about yourself emotionally correlates more readily with how you look than how you feel physically. In trying to lift your spirits emotionally by looking your best, you may not look like someone who is sick on an ongoing basis. It is really hard for others to understand that you don't feel well when you look well.

You may need to actually choose which part of yourself you want others to identify you by. A deliberate choice may need to be made to learn to separate how you feel physically from how you feel about yourself emotionally, so that your ill health doesn't cause emotional illness. Always emotionally projecting your illness image will affect your relationships. This will subsequently affect you emotionally and physically in a feedback loop manner. The ultimate response may be, "the body's a sick joke, but I'm doing great!"

How you feel about yourself is made up of many components. One of these is your sexuality. Awareness of your sexual identity so penetrates the fabric of adult life that you lose any consciousness of its presence (Money and Erhardt, 1967) until it is threatened or overshadowed by a new reality. The identity of a specific organic or psychiatric diagnosis can displace your sexual identity as male or female.

The prevailing identity of "I am illness" makes it difficult for you to relate to others from your former identity. This perpetuates further losses of relationships and cycles back into more grieving.

There may be times when you need to totally and honestly own your illness identity and neither cover up nor exaggerate it. Some of these occasions might be when you go to see your doctor, when in the hospital, when around understanding friends and family, or during times of increased disease activity when you are forced to "act sick" and need to depend on the aid of others to carry out your daily duties. There are also times when it is appropriate to play down your illness, but not in a way that totally denies it. It may take a long time to know where, when, and with whom to comfortably own your illness, and how much of it, when greeted with the question, "How are you?" Expect some "goofing up" and be easy on yourself when you do. Just try to learn from these times.

SUMMARY

You want to hold onto all you can from the life of health. Whether your looks become a blessing or a curse is all in the way you handle it. As your illness fluctuates, you may continue to struggle between whether or not to identify yourself only with your illness identity or with your total identity as a person, accentuating the positive. You can be the best-looking, sexy, sick person there ever was!

Understanding some of the dynamics of the question, "How are you?", identifying and utilizing your own special support persons, formulating some automatic, humorous responses, and absorbing the illness as only part of your total identity may be some ways of reducing the anger, bitterness, and loneliness possibly provoked in these frequent, casual brushes. You *can* become more relaxed in these situations as time passes. As you become more comfortable with yourself and your illness, others will be more at ease as well.

Don't forget to ask . . . "and how are things going with you?"

2

Relationships / Support Persons

When illness, tragedy, divorce, or any event in life occurs, producing change with a resulting grief process, many times your old emotional support systems may be rearranged, shattered, and disorganized. They may strengthen, becoming deeper and more meaningful than ever before. Also, you may notice those you had counted on before slowly and silently pulling away.

The person who becomes chronically ill or physically disabled experiences several types of real or imagined losses. The most important of these include loss of privacy, body image, and human relationships (Purtillo, 1976, p. 281). There may be much support at time of diagnosis or during a crisis, only for supportive relationships to taper off just when the patient is fully coming to grips with the reality of the situation, two or three months down the road.

The able-bodied may grow weary and possibly disillusioned by the ill person's inability to return to the real world of involvement, independence, and responsibility. Some may become angry when the ill person "refuses" to come home or return to work where he belongs.

"This tapering off of supportive relationships often is the most difficult loss the patient has to face in chronic illness. The friends and relatives who do not disappear out of neglect, exhaustion, or despair often become more dear" (Chyatte, 1979, p. 16).

"Some relatives and friends may react to your illness in a peculiar way. Their reactions vary according to their own problems and fears. Close friends may ignore you because they can't express their feelings. Some may be stoic and keep a stiff upper lip; some may become awkward and not know what to say; others may become overly concerned" (Chyatte, p. 15).

"It seems that when you fall ill and stay ill, people feel sorry for you. Sometimes, the sorrier they feel, the more it makes them feel vulnerable. They are afraid something serious will happen to them. They can't face you because they're so threatened by what has happened to you. Many people back off from what's strange and different, and let's face it, you are strange to other people; they've never experienced anything like what you've gone through" (Chyatte, p. 15).

At the same time, you may be pulling away from others, because you are uncomfortable with yourself, thereby creating a double "pull-away." No one goes through a problem alone. You take bystanders with you. You unwittingly victimize others as you go along. Mostly, you do not intend that it should be so, but under stress, your human reactions can normally, be pretty ugly. You are so busy acting defensively in your own behalf that you fail to see the wreckage around you (Ahlem, 1978, p. 62).

You may have to experience this shifting of your emotional support system while going through the toughest part of your grieving: the loss of life as it used to be. Understanding the dynamics of what's happening may release some of the inherent bitterness, allowing you to seek out a new support system. It may be that your best support persons will be those who have been touched by some grief that gives them the authentic ring of "having been there." Casual friends who have been sensitized by events in their own lives may be the ones who can reach out and be sustaining.

"People, by and large, will relate to the image you project. Friends will like you or dislike you according to what you do, what you say, and how you make them feel. If you project the image of a sick, dependent person, that's how you'll be treated" (Chyatte, p. 16).

Until you are comfortable with yourself, others can't be comfortable with you. It may take some education, self-examination, and counseling to get to the point where you are comfortable with yourself.

Normal relationships can be uncomfortable, as people may pity or feel sorry for the chronically ill person. Others may put you on a pedestal as being so wonderful for the way you handle things. Either approach is awkward to live with.

In reality, you are just like anyone else trying to cope with the many facets of living. It is only with time that you can "earn" the stance of just being an "average Joe", making it the best way you can.

From these general relationships, a few precious supportive relationships may emerge—those who can simply be there with you where you are, to share your hurts and pains or joy and victories. It may take time to discover who these people are, but they will slowly become apparent. Often, it may be up to you to take the first step, because people may not know how to react to you. Someone who has shared an experience or had similar experiences can more easily become a support person.

On the other hand, a genuine, sensitive, caring person with a knowledge of your background can become one of those among the ranks of the few. In some instances, in reaching out to be a support person for someone else, you may cultivate a support person for yourself.

Through trial-and-error, you may actually have to establish a grading process of receptivity levels of the people around you. Grade one are those who can hear the whole story. Grade two are those who can hear only a very condensed version. Grade three are those who only want an "I'm OK" or "I'm not so good." Grade four are those who only want to hear "everything is fine." This may take some time and people may shift back and forth between grades from time to time, depending on what's happening in their lives.

When you are hurting, you can suffer in an irresponsible, manipulative way. Complaining, moaning about your fate, making others feel guilty because they are not hurting or doing enough, placing excessive demands on your friends, or expecting people to do what can be done by yourself—all of these can lead to a helpless, self-pitying attitude. By shifting blame onto others, you, the sufferer, have found a way to avoid facing and doing something about your own problems (Collins, 1978, p. 149).

Ultimately, you alone are responsible for taking care of yourself: physically, emotionally, mentally, and spiritually. No one can do it for you. Others can only give encouragement and offer advice. The doctor, psychiatrist, pastor, family, and friends are only guides and supports. You have to do the real work yourself.

The first step toward emotional health is assuming responsibility for yourself. The second step is realizing you have to take care of yourself first before you can take care of anyone else. Any other commitments should come second or you will shortchange all involved, mainly yourself! Sometimes you need education and counseling to know how to take care of yourself best.

Even those special support persons may need a vacation from sharing problems when grappling with difficulties of their own. An honest sharing of feelings and a respect for the needs and schedules of others are much healthier. Support can and should be a two-way street to be healthy. It is important to be willing to help others when needed.

Once a person is identified as a support person, it does not mean he will be there forever. Your interests shift, lives take different directions, and contact may be lost. Some will hang in there. Don't put all your "eggs in one basket."

Your spouse or family members may not be able to support you at all or may be supportive only at times. If they can't do this, they can't. They need support, too, and need to be accepted where they are. They can't be forced or expected to be something they're unable to be. You may have to look elsewhere and spread the support out among several people. Supportive counseling may be needed.

At a time of diagnosis or crisis, you may need to talk incessantly about the illness and yourself in an exhibitionist manner. This need lessens with time, as the illness becomes an integrated part of your life rather than the main focus, and support lines are identified.

Your family and support persons may grow understandably weary during these times and may need more help than usual themselves. They have to juggle their own fears and uncertainties in addition to your needs, while still maintaining balance. They may fear failure and that they may not be able to go the distance. Everyone needs support persons in their lives, but those carrying special burdens, and significant others around them, need support in a more crucial way.

SUMMARY

"Silent suffering leads to the building of psychological barriers that keep other people out. Suffering alone can also be self-defeating. Without the objectivity, support, and encouragement of others who care, there is a tendency to withdraw into your own little world of self-pity, helplessness, and bitterness." (Collins, p. 148).

This would apply to your whole family, since your chronic illness affects each individual member of your family and the unit's functioning as a whole. As time passes, you'll find that those precious ones who are able to go the distance with you become rare treasures, and that the real wealth of this life is to be found in those relationships. Initiating and nurturing relationships may become your number one priority, as you are forced to slow down and "smell the roses of life."

3

It's "All in the Family"

The response of the family has great bearing on the ultimate adjustment, motivation, and expectations of a patient trying to cope and live with chronic illness. If you anticipate being included as a part of the functioning family unit, with as many of your former roles preserved as possible, you can be greatly influenced to engage in a treatment program. Your family unit and individual family roles may be altered and may have to be rebuilt along different priorities and guidelines, as ongoing illness becomes a part of your daily lives.

Adjustment to a chronic illness has to be a "family affair," not just your efforts. Stresses within you and your family have a rebounding effect that needs to be dealt with as a whole. With the sequential phases of chronic illness involving diagnosis, remission, flares and, finally, death, there are phase-related tasks that must be resolved. Failure to cope with one phase may jeopardize the total coping process of your family.

The success in handling any crisis depends on minimizing the time it takes to face the painful circumstances, comprehending (even hazily) what they mean, and moving on to life as it exists in the present. The loss of life as it used to be and anticipated losses in the future must be mourned as a family, finding comfort and solace in one another. Mourning may be experienced over a long period of time and may also be intermittent.

The initial task is squarely facing the diagnosis and all its meaning together. Denial, expressed by flights into activity such as a job change or move, shopping for a cure, hostility, change in family composition, travel, unnecessary expenditures—all are ineffective coping efforts and add to the burden to be carried by all.

Family members may take opposite sides, such as disagreeing on how to define the illness, who to discuss it with, and what to tell others about it.

Legitimate expectations under stress left unmet by family members may breed resentment and dissatisfaction, thereby decreasing the effectiveness of the joint effort essential for family coping.

Your extended family may or may not be able to participate and be helpful. Longstanding, unspoken jealousies and hostilities, power struggles, and negative family dynamics that have existed just below the surface may erupt into a full-blown family feud as you are diagnosed with a significant health problem. You and your nuclear family unit may have to serve as caretakers of the extended family.

Families may be more hurtful than helpful, as you may not be able to continue filling family roles you've filled in the past. The whole family structure as it once existed may have to shatter as old roles die, shift, and are reformed. This may not be all bad, since healthier patterns of relating may emerge. Some families may ultimately fall apart, while others grow closer and healthier due to the illness.

Communication lines with gut-level honesty need to be kept open for *all involved* to express their anger, hurt, and frustration. The family that cries, yells, and laughs together may stay together! Openly recognizing opposing coping positions may open the door to new ways of coping together.

Problems present in a marriage before the added stress of ongoing illness may have to be worked through before any progress can be made. Maintaining any meaningful relationship involves hard work. The addition of chronic illness to the picture may increase and intensify preexisting problems and create new ones. The need for hard work in the family becomes even greater.

Outside help may be needed to leap the hurdles, enabling you all to celebrate life together. Facing this possible need for help may be difficult to handle, but it is essential. Family therapy, group counseling, or individual counseling may provide the guidance needed to identify and accept things that need acceptance, or deal with and change things that need to be changed, in order to face life with chronic illness together as a family unit.

SUMMARY

When you are diagnosed with a chronic illness, you cannot be treated in isolation. Your pain, confusion, and distress will be registered in your family, too. Your whole family unit, with you as a member of that system, needs to be treated. The needs, feelings, problems, and resources of every member of the family must be taken into consideration.

Your illness may play a very important role within your family unit—reducing tension, giving unity of purpose, or providing identity. Until the role your illness plays in the family is understood, it may be treated in isolation from the dynamics that may have triggered it and serve to prolong it. You may be treating just the expression of or part of a problem when you treat the illness or the ill person in isolation from the family.

4

The Doctor / Patient Relationship

"We're getting married! We're going to be in this together for a long time—maybe the rest of your life. I'll be honest with you and I want you to be honest with me. If you don't like something or you disagree with me, please tell me. We'll work it out." This is the way an oncology (the study of tumors) surgeon, a friend of mine, starts out his relationship with each cancer patient.

One of the most important relationships a person with a chronic illness has is the doctor / patient relationship. It is much akin to a marriage, where there is a give-and-take, agreements and disagreements, some good and some bad. It is a relationship that needs to be worked at with honesty, concern, and respect by both parties. No doctor is perfect, as no patient is perfect. As with a marriage, personalities have to naturally blend to some degree. It takes two-way, gut-level communication.

Time is required to build a sound doctor / patient relationship. The relationship will be long-term, with the doctor's opinions and judgments reaching into many areas and decisions of the patient's life. Perhaps the patient is at his or her lowest physically and emotionally, or is frightened and confused when this "marriage" is initiated, hardly the best time to get "married."

Funny things can happen in the interaction between these two human beings. Feelings of anger related to the illness and loss of privacy may be displaced on the doctor, since there may be no other acceptable target for these feelings. The doctor may also displace feelings of frustration on the patient.

A power struggle may develop to establish who's "in charge." The doctor, who may be used to wielding a great deal of power, may find it difficult to relinquish some control to the patient, and vice versa. A working partnership is preferable.

What may be for the doctor just another fleeting moment in a long day of many patients may be a long-awaited and remembered "holy moment" for the patient, to be played and replayed over and over.

During this "holy moment," the whole direction of a life may be changed. A suspected diagnosis may be announced to "officialdom." Restrictions presenting many complicating factors may be officially recognized and sanctioned. The unknown may be clarified to produce greater unknowns.

The patient's level of anxiety may be so heightened that nothing is heard, much less understood or comprehended past the first five seconds or minutes. The patient's mind may go into orbit, not to return to earth or reality for some time to follow. The patient may need to go over and over the same material with the doctor on return visits, in order to absorb, understand, and deal with it all.

The doctor or patient may project his own emotions, motivations, and behaviors on the other. A patient looking for an authority figure may see the doctor as a "father-figure." Patients may fall in love, in a sense, with their doctors. Each may seek approval and affirmation from the other.

Sexuality plays an important part in all relationships, especially in the doctor / patient relationship, since it is of such an intimate, ongoing nature on many levels. The patient may want a closer, personal relationship. At the same time, the doctor may need his professional distance. All this undercurrent and more may be going on while transacting health care in a limited time frame. Quite a feat!

There must be an appropriate balance of dependence and independence at play. "The doctor appears God-like. He's your lifeline. There is no doctor who can keep you in good health. He can only tell you what you have to do" (Chyatte, 1979, p. 94). You need to learn to listen to the doctor as only part of your perspective, and also to listen to your body and interpret what it is saying, comparing the two interpretations. From this input, you formulate a plan of action.

Anger and hurt may be by-products of the emotionally charged medical arena. They may or may not be justified. In either case, they need to be confronted and appropriately vented. At times with a marriage, a divorce may be healthy, but only after momentous communication efforts fail to save it.

A change of doctors may also be necessary, but only after real efforts have been made to salvage the relationship. It is difficult to duplicate real-life events shared by a doctor and patient in a written or verbal report. Months or years may be spent cultivating a new partnership.

"Doctors and patients each have their special needs, and how these blend or collide inevitably has a bearing on the quality of health care" (Benet, 1979, p. XII). Doctors are human and experience physical, emotional, and spiritual problems, too. Doctors, in many cases, "lead lives no better integrated than those of the people they are employed to treat and sustain" (Benet, p. 150). This is evidenced by "psychological symptoms, severe marital problems and divorce, regular consultations with a psychiatrist, alcoholism, drug abuse, and suicide, seen in the doctor population" (Benet, p. 149).

The doctor has the continual pressure of making rapid, life-balancing decisions. Training has instilled the ideals of relieving suffering rather than helping people accept and learn how to best live with it. Confronting suffering they cannot relieve produces personal distress with which a doctor must cope.

Doctors may be caught in a double-bind situation. There may be anger or frustration if a patient doesn't improve. On the other hand, if the patient does improve, they may lose a relationship meaningful to them in subtle ways.

"Illness provides doctors with their livelihood, identity, and opportunities for distinction; illness causes patients to suffer. Doctors need patients just as patients need doctors. The relationship between them is intimate because they are both involved in their different ways with illness itself" (Benet, p. XII).

SUMMARY

"Some kind of partnership between doctor and patient is desirable and possible in all branches of clinical medicine" (Benet, p. 188). For this to happen, you, as the patient, need to assume responsibility for yourself.

Also, the doctor must relate in a way that allows you, as an equal partner, to assume an active role in your treatment. For a partnership of this nature to evolve, both participants need to display trust, honesty, respect, caring, and commitment to the workings of the relationship.

PART II

Relating to Yourself

5

Secrets . . . Present Moment Living

As you experience the journey through life, you stumble upon secrets of living that sustain you and make your task less of a burden. It seems that those who carry extra burdens in life, such as chronic illness, may out of necessity stumble more readily onto some of the secrets that enrich life, giving it greater meaning, and lightening their load.

Two secrets I have come across in my journey with chronic illness are present moment living and realistic hope. These became apparent at different stages along the way and continue to be clarified. Although they seem somewhat contradictory, they are both essential.

Fog engulfed me after I seemingly dropped off the end of the earth into an entirely new existence—and then was diagnosed. I found myself consumed with fear of what the future would hold, mourning and longing to have things back the way they were in the past.

Shadows of my new life began emerging, but I found myself imprisoned by the bars of yesterday and tomorrow. In a mere survival struggle, I found myself praying, "Give me this day my daily bread," trying desperately to focus on one day at a time—one moment at a time.

I found that it took intentional effort not to dwell on thoughts from the past and the future, but to concentrate on my todays. Taking one moment, one day at a time was more manageable. It set me free to enjoy and experience where I was.

I would slip back into my old patterns and have to will myself back to the day-by-day, moment-by-moment frame of mind. I realized that I couldn't control what thoughts came into my head, but I could control what I did with them. I could either dwell on them or deliberately block them out and focus on something else.

"One way to combat immobilization, however slight, is to learn to live in the present moment. Present moment living, getting in touch with your 'now,' is at the heart of effective living" (Dyer, 1976, p. 23). All we really have any certainty about is the present moment.

That precious moment is tarnished and wasted if you constantly invest your energies and hopes of living in the future—that future goal, that remission, or that magical time when things will get beter. The future can also loom ahead as a great, feared unknown.

Clinging to the glories, the hurts, the resentments, or the guilt from the past can also be confining. You have to live where you are, not where you used to be in the past—or hope to be in the future.

Victor Frankl, a Jewish psychiatrist who experienced life in a Nazi concentration camp, observed that many times you can't choose your circumstances, but you can choose what to do with those circumstances (Frankl, 1962, p. 66).

"The present moment, that elusive time which is always with you, can be most beautifully experienced if you allow yourself to get lost in it. Drink in all of every moment and tune out the past which is over and the future which will arrive in time. Seize the present moment as the only one you have" (Dyer, p. 24).

Slowly, present moment living evolved from a survival tactic to a means of celebration, and the ultimate in living and experiencing all of life, whether confined to bed or up and about, the abundant life. "The significance of life is not to be measured in terms of its length, but in terms of the depth of our days, the fullness, the totality, the wild, open abandon with which we give ourselves, day-by-day, to our days" (Raines, 1977, p. 83).

There is something of beauty and value in every moment, no matter what our situation—whether it be a relationship, an inner sense of peace and joy, the unending beauty and drama of nature, the sheer determination to stick things out, a total awareness of all about us, deciphering a doubt, or discovering a truth.

Ever so little by little—month by month and year by year—the grip of fear and mourning began to loose its death hold on my being so I could venture out into life and risk once again. "The coming future with its novelty and spontaneity outwits us always with its strange newness and unpredictable happenings, so that you need a deep confidence and flexibility of spirit enabling you to trust the process. You need to go with the flow and to use the light touch" (Raines, p. 141).

Gradually, I cautiously allowed myself to emerge from the cotton batting that I had wrapped myself in, as I waded back into life to test the waters. It was as though I needed some time wrapped in a cocoon, somewhat isolated, in order to emerge once again. Like the delicate winged butterfly, I ventured forth as a much changed creature—fragile but strong; more aware of myself, of life, and of others; knowing what it was to die to myself and then be reborn.

SUMMARY

I am still trying to learn how to totally experience and gently kiss the joy of my present moments, as if they were lightly floating butterflies, and to lovingly let them take their places in the past as others replace them. To cling too tightly to them would crush and destroy them. "To kiss the joy as it flies is to live in the Spirit; it is to live boldly, immediately with gracious abandon, daring to risk much, willing to give oneself. It is to live for a moment 'in unison with our dream'; to see the sun shining in the eyes of the smallest creatures; to create the marvelous by contagion" (Raines, p. 85).

6

Secrets . . . Hope

Live in the present—which is beautiful—and stretches beyond the limits of the past and the future. Present moment living started off as a survival tactic for me that evolved into a way to celebrate life. Striving to live in this mode became my hope, but then I realized that hope for present moment living wasn't enough. There had to be hope and goals that reached out into the future, too.

Hope can't be reasoned or bought. Once there, it cannot be swayed by logic or thought. Hope cannot be summoned up at will, but can survive the most difficult circumstances. As a small spark of light, it reaches out to the future, giving life meaning and direction.

Hope gives no guarantees, but gives strength and endurance. Hope has great power, as seen in the effects a placebo can have, when coupled with positive expectations, to produce relief from pain and even banish illness.

Hope can actually change the physiologic state of our bodies. "Feelings of hope and anticipation are recorded in the limbic system, messages are sent to the hypothalamus, reflecting the altered emotional state from hopelessness that includes the increased will to live. The hypothalamus then sends the messages to the pituitary gland that reflect the altered emotional state" (Simonton, 1978, p. 80). A chain reaction occurs, with hope as a catalyst, which results in a more healthy balance for your body.

"It is a peculiarity of man that he can only live by looking to the future. Those who know how close the connection is between the state of man—his courage, hope, or lack of them—and the state of immunity of his body, will understand that the sudden loss of hope can have a deadly effect" (Frankl, 1962, pp. 72, 75).

Hope must remain within the confines of reality, to some degree. Frankl observed that fellow concentration camp prisoners who set unrealistic deadlines for release withered and died when those dates came and passed without freedom.

Professionals in rehabilitation medicine know that goals set for the patient must be structured to introduce realistically attainable goals with increasing difficulty. If totally unrealistic goals are set and the patient fails, hope is dashed and future progress is hampered.

Attaining a realistic goal breeds hope for reaching out to more difficult ones. "Hope, then, is the ability to transcend what is and to be able to look at the experience as the pledge and first fruits of what is to be" (Werner-Beland, 1980, p. 187).

Realistic hope needs to encompass acceptance of what is without eliminating the possibility of what might be. "Creative hope involves recognizing your limitations and exploring your strengths. You may hope for more recovery, and also hope as you reach specific goals for yourself. Hope will grow as you recognize your own value. It is based on who you are, not on what you can do" (Cox-Gedmark, 1980, p. 30).

When reaching the adjustment phase in dealing with a crisis, you begin to feel the awakening of hope. Pockets of depression may remain and return at times, but the outlook is more positive. "The fact of the return of hope and positive expressions is a signal that the time for insight has returned. You are ready for an understanding of life in a new way." (Ahlem, 1978, p. 57). You may begin to reconstruct your life; gain new insights, appreciations, and concepts; set new goals; and be able to minister to others.

SUMMARY

Hope strangely began to emerge in my heart and mind from seemingly nowhere—almost like a bulb planted in the soil of the dark night of my being and soul—called forth by the promise of warmth and light. It was like experiencing the springtime of my soul, as new thoughts began to bud, new dreams were born, and new directions sprang forth in the perfect timing of the seasons of my life and living.

It was tempting to ignore, thwart, or crush these tender fragile, budding eruptions of promises of life. With them was an attendant threat of further disillusionment, lost dreams, failure, and pain. I could choose to argue away these tentative hope-thoughts or to listen to their whisperings of things to come and haltingly follow their calling one step at a time, finding my way beyond where I was.

At times I stumble, stagger, and lose my way, but determinedly, patiently, and tenaciously, day by week by month by year, I whistle in the dark and make slow, forward motion. One step leads to the next, and I am awed as I look back and see that my footprints in the sand have been leading somewhere and not just aimlessly wandering.

7

Grief in Chronic Illness

Grief is seen as natural and even expected in the loss of a loved one or "significant other." How much more intense and magnified does that grief become when the significant person being grieved is a part of you or of your being? Losses encountered by the chronically ill may not be quite as obvious as other losses to be grieved, but they nonetheless must be grieved appropriately and adequately in order to pick up the threads of present life . . . in the "now."

A great deal has been written about grief experienced in facing terminal illness. Very little has been written about grief in chronic illness, but some corollaries can be drawn from terminal illness. Elizabeth Kubler-Ross, in her book, *On Death and Dying*, makes a distinction between reactionary and preparatory depression in the grief process of the terminally ill.

In reactionary depression, the immediate losses and changes in life are grieved. In preparatory depression, the ultimate losses that are to come in death are grieved. The chronically ill must deal with both types of depression, but there is a greater emphasis on the reactionary grief.

Loss and change are normally a part of life. They may not be noticed much and are naturally absorbed into the lifestyle. Chronic illness may · accelerate the losses and label them in an undeniable way. "There are so many little dyings along the way that it doesn't matter which of them is death. When a patient is preparing for the acceptance of that final dying is closely related to the period following trauma or illness when the patient is preparing for adjustment to physical disability or chronic illness and the little dyings due to disabling illness or injury" (Purtillo, 1976, p. 280).

The big or small losses accumulated along the way in chronic illness result in a long-term grieving process that is influenced by the way the initial grief is handled. Among the things that may be lost by the chronically ill are health, fantasies of immortality, privacy, control, role identity, independence, means of productivity or self-fulfillment, self image, dreams or goals for the future, relationships, old ways of sexual expression, feeling good, undisturbed sleep, play or recreational activities, and energy, plus many other losses that serve as an expression of the self.

Purtillo (p. 281) postulates that, of these losses, privacy, body image, and relationships are the most important. "The tapering off of supportive relationships often is the most difficult reality the person has to face in either chronic or terminal illness" (pp. 281-82).

DIFFICULTIES IN THE GRIEF PROCESS

Grieving the losses in chronic illness has its own peculiar difficulties. "Perhaps one of the major differences between grief associated with long-term illness and disability and grief associated with the loss of a significant other is that the person is there to mourn his own loss" (Werner-Beland, 1980, p. 42). He is in attendance at his own small dyings.

"The person not only has his own burden, but he also feels the impact of others grieving for him and because of him. Resolution of grief in this instance must, by virtue of the fact that the source of grief is still present, involve all the principal characters in this life drama" (Werner-Beland, p. 42).

After reacting to a diagnosis of chronic illness, your family faces a period of redefining its situation as a family. In the process of realization, your famiy needs to examine its "old" family view of the world and to formulate a "new" family view. This process is much like the way you synthesize and incorporate a new self identity as part of your new, accepted, self-awareness (Lewis, 1983, p. 194).

It is a process where your family "gives up" its previous premorbid or preillness identity and formulates a new image. In coming to terms with themselves, family members become something other than what they were. This process of renegotiating and reformulating your new family image with accompanying role fluctuations is a major transition.

The process of "becoming" is a turbulent, ongoing, back and forth, difficult process. Through experience, your family, as a system, needs to come to an understanding of how its meaningful relationships are affected by your altered capacity to sustain your previously designated roles and functions within the family system (Werner-Beland, 1980, p. 53).

You and your family may go through the grief process at different paces. If all involved don't have a firm sense of their own personhoods, you may get stuck in the anger, bargaining, and depression without letting go of the old life to move into the present. You may cling to remnants of the old, highly valued memories of what your family used to be like and those unrealistic, mythical expectations of what your family should be.

You and your family may get caught in a cyclical pattern of grieving and searching for the lost way of life, and never make it through the grief to acceptance. There may be an attempt to superimpose the old life on top of the "now," giving a false sense of having made it through the grief process. This will only work for a time, until your pretense can no longer be maintained and the pain becomes intense and unbearable.

Family members may not understand their continued mood swings and grieving behaviors. All of you may become impatient with one another in your different stages of the grieving process. "The end result may be a build-up of tension between you and other members of the family . . ." (Werner-Beland, p. 37).

Your grieving process may be thwarted by anger, poor communication, and denial. Anger in the grief process "hooks" into the eternal "why" that rings against the sky. Resolution would be easier if a cause or reason could be pinpointed, allowing closure. An answer may not be found and may have to be left unanswered.

Added to this anger may be anger that arises from long–standing resentments, interfamily control issues, or anger from past wrongs. There is no appropriate place to vent or direct this anger. It may be directed within your family, causing more anger to multiply. With chronic illness your sources of anger may multiply, making anger pervasive in the family.

Poor communication may show up in different members of your family. They may take immovable, differing points of view on almost anything and everything related to the illness. Poor communication prevents grieving, weakens and undermines your family relationships, facilitates denial, and encourages behaviors that foster avoiding the real problem.

Denial may be seen in your getting caught up in every activity available, and is accompanied by the inability of you, your family, or both to face the realities of your illness and to grieve. A change in family make up, buying a new home, a sudden urge to get a new job, foolishly spending money, and traveling may all be signs of denial. All these things further support denial, increase your family's burdens, and absorb both physical and emotional resources needed to deal with the illness.

If the losses occur at a time of important tasks and when there is a need to maintain the morale of others grieving those same losses, you may show little or no reactions for weeks or even much longer. In addition, with a phasic illness that has a tendency to come and go, such as MS, SLE, or rheumatoid arthritis, the necessity of grieving may be easily denied. During times of feeling better, the illness may be completely denied. In worsened health, you may be overwhelmed by despair and be hypersensitive and acutely aware of your illness (Shontz, 1975, p. 85).

NECESSITY FOR GRIEVING

Delayed grief may result in maladaptive behaviors such as severe reactions to separation, unexplained somatic responses, specific medical diseases, altered relationships with your friends, relatives, and others (Lindeman, 1965, p. 13). An intellectual as well as an emotional process has to be worked through.

The intellectual process may proceed and pave the way for the emotional, gut-level, heart-rending emotional process. It may take some time living with the chronic illness to actually determine the losses that need to be grieved.

Overintellectualization by itself may serve as a form of denial, keeping a distance from the pain of the emotions. "Depression and tears seem to be the mechanism that restores the grieved to normalcy" (Chyatte, 1979, p. 10). The grieving seems to lance the emotional wounds, allowing anger, bitterness, hurt, and disappointment to be released in this letting-go process of what used to be. Without grieving, these emotional wounds may produce more handicapping effects than the illness itself.

Physiologic changes due to chronic illness, depression, and the grief process all, individually and together, have the potential of producing emotional responses that would perpetuate grief into a cycle if they were not resolved. Inactivity from lack of motivation, secondary to not feeling well emotionally or physically, progressively inhibits the functioning of the part of the nervous system that automatically controls physical balance in the body.

The blood circulates more slowly, the poisons in the blood are not cleansed away, and the system becomes sluggish. When this happens, the physical symptoms of the depressed state tend to increase, and thence the physical supplements the emotional in terms of the downward spiral of organic states (Jackson, 1977, p. 64).

There is a need to work through the "grief so that one can get the past in perspective and find meaning in the present" (Cox-Gedmark, 1980, p. 21). This also requires developing coping strategies to help make the most of what is in the "now." "Grieving the loss entails a progression from the initial reaction of numbness of disbelief to a growing awareness of pain, sorrow, and often anger and preoccupation with the lost object, and gradually reorientation in which the loss is accepted and equilibrium restored" (Moss, 1977, p. 18). Certainly, to deal with chronic illness successfully, you need to work through the grief process and its stages. Rebuilding life in the present is impossible until the past is relinquished.

BENEFITS OF GRIEVING

Grieving the loss of the old you, in the world of the healthy, may give birth to the new you, in the "now." In this process, you may find the essence of your own individual worth not overshadowed by or enmeshed in the peripheral aspects of living and constant doing. Interests and talents there was once no time for the in the past may emerge, to be cultivated in the present.

New strengths may develop as by-products of coping with chronic illness. The gift of life, without conditions, may be more deeply treasured and celebrated. You may become aware that you are a *whole person*, even in the midst of chronic illness.

Grief may be awakened in times of increased disease activity of your chronic illness or other additional illnesses, additional losses, during the anniversary of a loss or other special days, and times of crisis. This grief may be more easily handled if there has been adequate grieving in the initial stages. Recent studies indicate that the healing process following significant loss takes longer than once thought, possibly two to four years (Melges-Demaso, 1980, p. 51).

Grief has to be experienced on your own timetable. It can't be pushed. As healing occurs, scar tissue may remain, making you even stronger. Scar tissue is stronger than tissue in its normal state.

Joy can replace sorrow, laughter can push aside the tears, peace can pervade turmoil, and involvement with life can appear in place of loneliness, as grief serves as a bridge between life in the past and life in the "now."

SUMMARY

You need to pay your tolls as you go along on the road of life. If you've run through or around toll gates along the way without paying the price, you'll find a road block somewhere along the way that may be impassable. The fine you'll have to pay at that point could shatter you. It may be very difficult and painful to find your way again.

Grieving is painful and difficult to face. You may try to avoid the grieving at all costs. The price you'll end up paying by avoiding the grief / pain process will be far more costly than the price you pay if you take all of life—the good and the bad, the enjoyment and the pain, the laughter and the tears, the peace and the anger, the acceptance and the grief—experiencing it to its fullest extent. The good and the bad taken together can become the best when you place your trust in the Spirit to redeem it all in His perfect grace and timing.

8

Keys to Grieving

In facing the pain of grieving, there may be the temptation to run away from the losses. "Man's tasks to fill up his emptiness and release his pain is the test of his character. His quick solutions through drugs, travel, or hard work can be as unreal as a romance immediately following the funeral" (Madden, 1970, p. 108). "When you try to block out the hurt and refuse to feel, you may cause your inner wounds to fester" (Cox-Gedmark, 1980, p. 14).

The pain and struggle a butterfuly must experience to gain freedom from its coccoon is the very mechanism that pumps the blood from its ungainly, engorged body to its wings, giving birth to a creature of delicate beauty. Without that struggle, the butterfly would emerge as a freak with a huge body and withered wings incapable of flight.

Key One: You have to stay with the pain and experience it in order to work through it.

Tears and courage are not opposites of each other. As a matter of fact, they are closely related. To be yourself, allowing your feelings to come out, is to be courageous. Tears won't change the outward circumstances, but they will change you. Tears allow the venting and release of emotions and may bring a new outlook to your life.

Key Two: Experience the pain and then let it go. You must let the tears flow to cleanse the wounds of grief, thereby allowing healing.

"Laughter, fun, and celebration are important aspects of life. They can help you keep your illness in perspective" (Cox-Gedmark, p. 54). "Grief and humor are often bound together because of the depth of the human problem and the desperate need to find some way of coping with it.

Humor reduces life's problems to the extent that they can be approached—first in humor, then in seriousness" (Jackson, 1977, p. 42). Basically, the same muscle systems are used in both laughing and crying. Both bring relief from tension.

Key Three: Learn to laugh, try to see humor in your situation, and celebrate life.

Facing and labeling your feelings and emotions, and the emotions of those around you, helps in honestly communicating with those significant persons closest and dearest to you—family, friends, doctor. This communication lets them know what they can do to help you. Communication with others helps to bear the load, reflect reality, and keep you on course. A burden shared is divided—a joy shared is multiplied.

Key Four: Keep the lines of communication open.

Some people deal with the pain of their grief by totally withdrawing. Others respond with panic in being alone at all. "When persons—through some false pride or privacy—seek to separate themselves from their loving community, the more quickly they sentence themselves to painful destructive expressions of their loneliness" (Jackson, p. 85).

On the other hand, being alone can provide a center of quietness from which calm, wise judgments, opportunities for personal growth, and creativity in living can emerge.

Key Five: Times of solitude and times of fellowship need to be alternated.

Sometimes, in being so close to the problems at hand, you may not be able to find your way through them on your own. You may be able to see the pieces of the puzzle clearly, but may not know how to fit them together. Anger and depression in the grief process may get so heavy that you can't pull the load on your own.

Key Six: You need to utilize your special support persons and seek counseling to help find the way.

Those who seem to be the most angry tend to see themselves as victims and not as participants in what has happened to them. Assuming responsibility for yourself is essential in mediating anger in the grief process.

Key Seven: Take responsibility for yourself and realize that you *do* play a role in your illness.

Faith is essential in stretching yourself beyond where you are. "When you allow God to be God, you're free to put the various aspects of your life in perspective and recognize other values. God is not a God who is 'out there.' God is within you, seeking to join with you in giving your life meaning and worth" (Cox-Gedmark, p. 114).

Key Eight: Faith gives hope and courage to reach beyond where you are and venture into the unknown.

Elizabeth Kubler-Ross describes five stages in the grief process. The final stage of acceptance in terminal illness is portrayed as a turning to the wall, separating one's self from life, a void of feelings, and preparing for death.

Acceptance of chronic illness needs to include dealing squarely with the little dyings and the threat of ultimate death. Rather than turning to the wall away from life, you have to grieve your losses in order to return *to* life.

Key Nine: In some ways, dying is the easy part—fully living presents the greater challenge. Death is merely a breathing out of the spirit, requiring no effort or energy, but only a release.

Sometimes adjustment is the word used when referring to living with a chronic illness, and acceptance used in reference to terminal illness. Both words can be summed up in the word "acknowledgement"—"assessing the losses that are to be incurred as a result of the illness, finding the uniqueness of the experience and facing it squarely, and the search for meaning in the experience" (Purtillo, 1976, p. 283).

"The chronically ill, more than others, need to come to terms with death" (Krupp, 1976, p. 122). Even though everyone is going to die, regardless of the cause, fear of death is one of the basic and most powerful human emotions. Dying is something everyone does in somewhat the same manner, but fear of death is ingrained from early childhood on. All of nature is constantly in a flux of life and death. Every seven years we become totally new beings, with every cell in our bodies having died and been replaced.

Key Ten: Our uniqueness comes in our living, not in our dying.

SUMMARY

"There is birth and death in every moment. Something is, and something else can never be again" (Powell, 1978, p. 50). It is not until you have come to terms with your own small dyings and ultimate death, embraced their reality, and found peace that you can be completely in touch with and embrace life and living. To deny death gives you only a partial view of life. To fearfully and frantically clasp life in your grip only squeezes the living out of it.

Focusing on the fear of death, or desperately avoiding it, blurs your vision of life, saps what energy there might be for living, and imprisons you in the future. You can't live in the present and enjoy life.

Living with a chronic illness may "scare you to death" in that you give up living to the fullest. The lyrics of one verse of the song, *The Rose*, are quite appropriate here:

> *It's the heart afraid of breaking that never learns to dance.*
> *It's the dream afraid of waking that never takes a chance.*
> *It's the one who won't be taken who cannot seem to give.*
> *It's the soul afraid of dying that never learns to live.**

Chronic illness has been known to shorten life expectancies. Therefore, it seems foolish to squander any of that precious gift.

Life must be experienced with a light touch, as a momentary gift. Otherwise, you end up stifling it, clinging too tightly in anxiety and fear. Daredevils feel a great exhilaration as they tempt death with death-defying feats. The person with a chronic illness can be equally daring, if he daily chooses to live life to the fullest, experiencing the same kind of exhilaration. This in no way means taking foolish risks with that precious gift.

As you have lived you will die. What you will become in the end will be more of what you are deciding and trying to be right now (Powell, p. 16). A roller coaster ride is much more painful and less enjoyable when you're frantically holding on. Relaxing, throwing your hands up, yelling and screaming at the top of your lungs in enjoyment—these give you a much more thrilling ride.

It may seem strange to be focusing on grief and death during the Christmas season, when many are rejoicing in the birth of the Christ child. Yet, it is only in the context of the meaning of Christ's death that His birth can be truly celebrated. He taught us how to live the abundant life and how to find victory in death. He showed us that it is the quality, not the length, of life that counts.

Eternity begins now, at this very moment. "Eternity is not permanence, but significance; not duration, but depth" (Raines, 1977, p. 83). Whatever your faith, may you find a new way of living that faces death squarely, then turns full face to life, rejoicing in the celebration of the gift of that life.

9

Living with Chronic Illness: Dying Is the Easy Part

Being a visiting nurse, active in my career and moving up the promotional rungs, hoping to get my nurse practitioner degree, and to do some innovative things in the home nursing field, I was suddenly knocked off my feet by health problems. Over a period of several months, I was diagnosed as having a chronic, phasic, incurable illness that could be fatal. Hearing the diagnosis over the phone late one Friday afternoon was like hearing a deafening gunshot in my ears, which echoed over and over.

My old lifestyle of work, activity, being athletic, singing as a soloist or choir member, church and community involvements, my roles of on-the-go mother and wife—"the Enjoli woman," who can take on any task and still be sexy at the end of the day—dimmed and faded from view as I fell deeper and deeper into a hole. I've never completely been able to crawl back out of it.

For a long while, I was able to deny the long-term consequences of my condition, since my illness held the possibility of remission somewhere on the horizon. Disease activity would also fluctuate from time to time. During brief reprieves of feeling slightly better, my spirits would soar, only to be dashed as the pain, fatigue, nausea, and other problems inevitably returned. Days stretched into weeks, weeks into months, and months into years.

My family and I kept taking the "old me" off the shelf, hoping one day she might return and we could go back to our past lives. We'd sigh and put her back on the shelf, but she lingered in our memories and hopes, thwarting any attempts of accepting and living in the present as it was. It was always, "Tomorrow we'll . . ." or "Remember yesterday, when . . . ?"

An article in a rehabilitation magazine comparing the multitude of small deaths from chronic illness and disability to ultimate death, and the grieving inherent in each, put a label on the emotions I was experiencing: grief and its stages of denial, bargaining, anger, depression, and acceptance. The writer pointed out that the accumulation of these small deaths caused ultimate death to pale in comparison.

Ultimately, grieving my losses served as a bridge allowing me to celebrate my todays to the fullest, instead of being imprisoned in my yesterdays or tomorrows. Recognizing that grief was appropriate and even necessary gave me the key to the door of my adjustment process.

LOSSES GRIEVED

I slowly began to realize the enormity of what I had relinquished in my living and what had ultimately died. This included my former good health; independence; sense of control; privacy; modesty; body image; relationships as they had been; self-image; established roles inside and outside the family; former social status; a sense of self-confidence; financial security; a means of productivity and self-fulfillment in work, at home, or in the community; lifestyle; plans and dreams for the future; the fantasy of immortality; familiar daily routines; undisturbed sleep; feeling good; many modes of expressing my sexuality; leisure activities—the list could go on and on.

Sense of Control Over Life

The sense that I had control over my body and life was shattered, leaving me extremely vulnerable. I would feel okay one minute and lousy the next. I was living in a body that had become a stranger, and seemed to continually change. I couldn't trust it anymore nor predict how it would respond to the demands I made on it.

I used to plan my life years in advance. Now it was difficult to make plans for even the next day, much less the future. Every day I gave up new controls over my body and emotions, taking medication to help endure the effects of the disease activity. The medication would add its own strange effects, causing an even greater sense of loss of control and helplessness.

Fear of the illness itself, with its many unknowns, created a greater sense of loss of control. Often, in searching for and finding no visible means of control, the sense of helplessness would bring on depression, adding to the depression that is sometimes part of the illness itself.

In his writings, Victor Frankl compares the loss of control in a prison setting to that of a person imprisoned in his body by chronic illness. I found, as he did in his prison experience, that I could control my attitude, even if I couldn't control my circumstances.

I could let fear, anger, or despair control me. On the other hand, I could accept responsibility for myself and choose to kiss the joy of each moment, tenderly caressing it and living it to the fullest, letting it go, and then turn to the next.

Sexuality

My grieving, as well as my illness, brought about changes in my means of sexual expression, response cycle, arousal, and feelings of sexuality. Sometimes it almost seemed like my illness identity threatened to replace my sexual identity. Ways in which I expressed and reinforced my sexuality, such as wearing high heels; dyeing and styling my long hair; walking a certain way; wearing flimsy negligees; getting a sexy tan in a bikini; going barefoot; wearing short shorts, short sleeves and sleeveless tops in the summer; dancing cheek to cheek; and other things had to be altered.

Putting on my cervical collar and "clod-hopper" orthopedic shoes did little to heighten my sense of sexiness. Fatigue and pain didn't provide feelings conducive to sexual arousal and encounter. In some ways, grieving the vanity losses connected with sexuality were some of the most difficult.

Changes in my lifestyle, such as employment, avocations, recreation, social life, economics, and living arrangements, all had direct effects on my sexual life, since sexuality is an expression of the total being. Sleeping habits at home had to be changed, and later a hospital bed invaded the bedroom. There were also times away during hospitalizations. Family roles that defined sexuality roles had to flip-flop as disease activity fluctuated.

With all these changes taking place in our lives, my husband and I found out anew how essential communication is in a sexual relationship.

In this way, assumptions are not erroneously made by one partner about the illness process that may drift into a way of life that isn't necessary. I have had to find new ways of expressing and heightening my sexuality, sexual expression, sexual arousal, and response that are possibly more fulfilling than they have ever been.

Productivity

I think the loss of my career is one of the ongoing and most agonizing areas of my life to grieve and let go of. My career was an extension of who I was and what I valued about myself.

To the pain of this loss was added the pain of the official Social Security disability decree that came after a year and a half of obstacles, red tape, financial disaster, confusion, questions, and doubts. This loss removed one of the most important means of control in my life.

Gone was my means of productivity, self-expression, self-fulfillment, social outlet, necessary financial support, means of identification, and lifetime investment. At the same time, I had to begin relating to a different end of the financial structure, with all the red tape, long waits, and humiliation of asking instead of giving. I had to contend with yet another identity and label—disabled—and all its societal and personal connotations.

My avocational loves of singing, church involvements, outdoor activities and athletics came as equally difficult areas to give up. In some ways, these avocations had greater meaning than my primary job, because they were interests I had pursued or been involved in since childhood.

Many of the avocations that were forfeited were activities that I had shared with my family, such as camping, and vacations, which cemented us together as a family. We had to grieve these losses together, large portions of our old lives vanished.

I had to find the value of my being, devoid of doing and the peripheral things of life, discovering new ways of self-expression that reached out to others, incorporating my illness and disability identities as only a part of my total being, and discerning new ways to be a part of my family and community. New identities that have emerged are free-lance writer, chaplain, counseling student, and an acceptance of myself, warts and all.

DIFFICULTIES IN
GRIEVING LOSSES

Grieving these losses was especially difficult for many reasons. Perhaps it was even more difficult than grieving the loss of a loved one. It was as if I was in attendance at my own small dyings, but there was no funeral to mark the end of it all, with the grieved object buried and out of sight.

While trying to grieve my own losses, I had to deal with all the varied responses of those around me who were also grieving: those who pulled away, overwhelmed; those who denied the need to grieve; those who wept openly over me; those who treated me as someone strange; and those dear ones who shared it all with me, at my own pace.

There was no end in sight, no closure, which made it even more difficult for those special support people to grieve their losses, go the distance, and not doubt their ability to endure whatever came. It took me almost two years to realize that what was gone was gone for good.

When I did realize the need to grieve and what needed grieving, the grief process would have to be stifled in order to confront important tasks at hand or to maintain the morale of those around me.

NECESSITY AND BENEFITS
OF GRIEVING

Until I actively mourned on an emotional and intellectual level the death of the person that I once was, celebrated what her life had been, and let her go, I could not fully love and accept the person I had become and celebrate her uniqueness.

Many relationships that had been ruptured as people pulled away from me in fear and as I pulled away in confusion, fear and hurt, could not heal and mend until grief had been lanced from my wounds and washed away by my tears.

Grieving helped me to get my past in perspective, instead of dwelling on it or the future, so that I could develop coping strategies to make the most of the present. My emotional well-being no longer depended on my physical well-being. My body could be falling apart, but my spirit could soar to new heights that I never knew were possible.

As I reached the acceptance stage in the grief process, joy slowly replaced sorrow, laughter pushed aside the tears, peace pervaded the turmoil, and involvement in life wherever I was appeared in place of loneliness. My grief will be reawakened with intercurrent illness, additional losses, anniversaries of losses, new crises, and at holiday seasons. My initial grieving, however, will make these times a little less devastating. By grieving my losses adequately, I will have a better chance of preventing emotional illness and other physical illness due to delayed grief, in addition to my present condition.

Along with grieving my small dyings, I have had to face the anticipatory grief of my ultimate dying. Accepting a terminal illness may be signaled when a person turns to the wall, cuts the ties to life, and withdraws from life and those in it, in resignation.

In chronic illness, I have had to grieve my daily and ultimate dyings. Acceptance is signaled as I try to return to fully living to establish new relationships and reestablish old ones as a different person, assume responsibility for myself, and resume life in an altered way.

SUMMARY

I have come to feel that dying is the easy part, the breathing out of the spirit, for it requires no effort. The real challenge lies in grieving my losses and then turning back to a life complicated by chronic illness, rejoicing in the daily celebration of the gift of that life—the joy-dance of present moment living!

10

Anger!

All emotions serve some purpose in the psychological make-up of a person. Emotions can be used in positive or negative ways, in healthy or unhealthy ways. Anger is one of the most misused, misunderstood, but most valuable emotions that exists in one's repertoire of emotions.

Unlike other emotions, anger has no pay-offs, but can actually control you, causing physical decline and cutting you off from significant others. Properly identified, labeled, and handled, anger can be an important means of communication within the self that needs venting to others.

By understanding anger, you can gain better control of it and be free to live a life of caring and concern, instead of letting it control you. Proper recognition, understanding, and channeling of this ever-present emotion can change your entire way of life, making it more comfortable and productive.

"Anger is a part of life. The question is whether it will be used to become more destructive of self and others, or whether it can lead to creative insight and useful action" (Jackson, 1977, p. 19). Anger can make you stubborn and unrealistic, create havoc in your life, or lead to better understanding of the self and reality.

WHAT IS ANGER?

Popular theories state that anger is a reaction to repressed childhood experiences, a frenzied style of crying out for love, the most extreme example of selfishness. None of these descriptions is totally correct, but there is a common thread in each. When anger comes into your life, it is usually

51

when you feel unappreciated, belittled, taken for granted, helpless, or in some way insignificant (Carter, 1983, p. 27), or when there is a form of frustration.

Anger is an immobilizing reaction, triggered when any expectation is not met. It is the result of wishing the world and people in it were different (Dyer, 1976, p. 210). When you are angry you do not allow for variety, but depend on and demand that life (the people and events in it) be a certain, prescribed way. You don't assume responsibility for yourself. The external, physical world controls your internal, emotional world.

Anger that is used to assertively speak up for and communicate personal needs, while also considering the needs of others, indicates a real strength. Selfishness can turn this constructive type of anger into a destructive, aggressive communication tool that "never works in changing others; it only intensifies the other's desire to control the angry person" (Dyer, p. 211). The way you use anger is what makes it either a bridge for communication or a wall shutting out communication.

Ideally, anger is a tool to help build relationships. In its pure form, anger is an emotional signal that tells you something needs to be changed. "It was intended to be a positive motivator to be used in giving one another feedback about how life can be lived more productively" (Carter, p. 35). What may need to be changed may be your expectations of life, your unreasonable dependence on others, events in life that meet your needs and make you happy, or the way you communicate with others.

CHRONIC ILLNESS
AND ANGER

Sources of Anger

Chronic illness is certainly not what you would expect or want to be a part of your life. With chronic illness, your expectations of what your life was to be like may be totally shattered and replaced by something that you would never have dreamed of.

At the same time, the expectations of significant others are also blown apart, creating anger in all involved in your life. As chronic illness invades your life, the things that trigger your anger may change and multiply.

Delay in diagnosis may initiate anger due to the frustration of looking for answers and not finding them. Anger may be stirred when medical health professionals can't offer assurances that everything will be alright; when they don't have all the answers; when there may be no remedy to relieve every ache and pain; when there may be no known cause, treatment, cure, or prognosis for an illness; or when medical bills mount up as the illness continues on a daily basis. "The family, as well as the patient, will experience anger, betrayal, and guilt over their loss of control as the results of ill health" (Werner-Beland, 1980. p. 98).

Anger tends to be one stage in the complicated passage of grief. Grief is a common and essential process in the adjustment to chronic illness. When you continue to grieve, you choose to unconsciously turn the stage of anger against yourself and others as part of your refusal to acknowledge the losses of self that are so attached to your being. In doing this, you do "not allow yourself to experience life in a real sense" (Werner-Beland, p. 173). You give up hope, living in a state of aggressive self-complacency (Marcel, 1962, p. 33).

Anger may be evoked by healthy people, since they are a reminder of what has been lost. Healthy people handling minor health problems in an irresponsible, complaining manner may cause you to steam. The chronically ill may have to suffer silently, sharing their trials with only a "special few."

The inability of the "crowd" to "listen" may provoke anger. Fear of losing the support of significant others and your ability to function may generate anger. The need for others to deny your illness can be maddening—"You *look* so good!"

A sense of hopelessness, helplessness, fear, and/or betrayal by the body adds yet additional logs to fuel the flames of anger. Limitations enforced by illness produce frustration and anger when they interfere with desired activities, and necessitate dependency on others for many things.

There may also be resentment and anger on the part of the person who has your dependency needs thrust on him. You may experience more anger and frustration when only marginally ill than when severely ill, since you may have one foot in the world of the healthy and one foot in the world of the sick. You can't be totally in either world.

Initially, anger may be caused by interference from well-meaning helpers. Their efforts to help may seem demeaning and be interpreted as pity or a lack of confidence in your ability to handle things on your own. Later on, when you are tired and need help, it may not be offered. Anger may brew because others may not be sensitive enough to recognize your need for help. You'd rather it be given without having to ask, since this is also demeaning.

Anger can be born from all these unique things that go with chronic illness, adding to the accumulation of the normal, everyday frustrations that hook into life-producing anger. When already angry, you tend to have a short fuse that causes anger to be set off more easily. Feeling ill doesn't make you the most cheerful person in the world, anyway! If you are chronically ill, you can expect to be angry from time to time.

Responses to Anger

"Some sick people turn anger outward, blaming others for their illness or for their failure to improve. Others turn inward, blaming themselves for their condition and feeling guilty because they cause themselves and others so much trouble and expense" (Shontz, 1975, p. 146).

"Pathological symptoms of repressed anger associated with unresolved or unwisely managed grief may show up in social behavior, changes in psychological patterns, or types of organic acting out that we recognize as illness. Skin rashes and hypertension are two examples" (Jackson, p. 16).

Another type of response is seen in attempts to assign blame by going over memories of events leading up to diagnosis. Presumably, if blame or responsibility could be assigned to someone or some event, what has happened might be undone. Resolution is easier if you can find a cause that would permit you to go on to closure.

Finding some reason or being able to put the blame for events on something or someone may be easier to live with than the realization that life is uncertain, that there are no guarantees, that many things can't be changed and must be lived with. Possible rationalized targets might be the doctor, a family member, or a poor diet. You may also try to explain your illness by mentally linking mysterious, irrational events, or not finding just the right formula of things to do.

Outlets for anger may be altered by chronic illness. Releasing anger's tension through jogging, walking, swimming, or any physical activity, may not be feasible anymore. The loss of these former outlets for physical tension may evoke even greater anger. New ways of tension release may have to be sought out and established in a trial–and–error fashion. What releases tension for one person may not for another.

The presence of chronic illness can provoke a great deal of anger in all affected by it: patient, family, and professionals. There is no suitable, tangible target to vent that anger on. Health care professionals often become the targets of this anger, since they are the closest at hand, the ones who pronounced the diagnosis, and a constant reminder of the illness that requires reliance and dependence on them for maintaining any semblance of well-being. Anger may be directed toward God, institutions, friends, family, and self.

Anger is a way of saying, "Notice my needs." Feelings of anger and irritability are displaced on those closest to you. Family and friends may experience similar emotions. While trying not to express these feelings directly to the patient, they may unconsciously direct as much anger toward the ill person (for getting ill and causing them inconvenience and pain) as they do toward themselves.

Anxiety of a spouse or other family member involved in the care of the patient may cause anger and hostility to build between them. A struggle to show who's in charge or in control may develop.

Anger is a common response to separation and loss. Initially, dysfunctional anger often accompanies physical illness or disability. This is because, at first, there is a sense of disbelief that the losses of the self and others are permanent. As permanence becomes a reality, anger is an attempt to signal the return of what is lost.

In illness, anger won't serve this function. Angry, aggressive behavior tends to alienate and drive significant others away, rather than bring them closer. When suffering loss frequently, your anger may seem selfish, unfeeling, irrational, out of proportion, and misdirected. Yet, this is understandable.

The person in the early phase of chronic illness frequently questions his own worth. "He wants people to be close and reassure him that they still like him and need him, even if he is sick. But the anger, whose aim is to signal the lost part or function to return, works against the formation or continuation of essential human relationships" (Werner-Beland, p. 23).

Within relationships, an anger/guilt/depression cycle may evolve. You may feel guilty and depressed because of your anger and angry over your guilt and depression, causing the whole situation to be controlled by anger.

"Your feelings cannot be ignored. If you don't deal with them, they will come out in other ways, perhaps with manipulative silence or excessive demands" (Cox-Gedmark, p. 47). Always being compliant and agreeable may stem from fear of expressing anger, but eventually the anger will either come out in your behavior or, worse, show up negatively in your health.

You don't go through a problem alone. You take those nearby with you. Others are victimized as you go along. You really don't intend for this to occur but, under stress, human reactions can be pretty ugly. When busy acting defensively in your own behalf, you can't see the damage you are doing to others around you (Ahlem, 1978, p. 62).

In accepting chronic illness, the anger should become less pervasive. A time of reconciliation and reconstruction may have to occur, as new realities are tested out and relationships mended. You are more at peace with yourself: as a result, you are at peace with those around you.

WAYS TO HANDLE ANGER

"There is no one correct way to handle anger. Obviously, the cir-cumstances are going to have an influence on how one chooses to deal with anger. There are three general styles in which people can handle anger: repression, expression, and release" (Carter, p. 93). Each style con-tains its own pitfalls and dangers that must be looked at and understood.

Repression of Anger

Repression of anger may result from fear of alienating significant others, or as a form of denial. You may feel that the anger, if not expressed, will go away. In denying anger, there is no obligation to deal with it. Repressed anger can be dangerous, since it can fester and grow in the subconscious, becoming especially powerful and bitter. Since anger is pushed into the subconscious, it is actually out of your immediate control. Excessive irritability and quarreling may result from repressed anger.

Expressions of Anger

Anger can be expressed in many ways, both verbally and nonverbally. Much anger may be expressed in passive-aggressive ways that tend to cut off any means of healthy, open, and honest communication. Anger may be seen in passive resistance to treatment and measures to improve your health. Somehow, you just can't follow that medication, diet, rest, or exercise regimen.

Doctor-shopping may be a sign of repressed anger that has resulted from not finding a doctor who will agree with you. Sarcasm is an indication of anger beneath the surface. Chronic complaining may spring from hidden hostility. Stubbornness may be a means of holding onto anger giving you a sense of power over others. Constant criticism of others reflects anger, an inadequacy in accepting life's imperfections, and a desperate attempt to shift the focus away from your own weaknesses. Chronic pain may elicit aggressive, hostile behaviors, and complaining can be an expression of masked anger.

Silence can be a potent expression of passive-aggressive anger, and is perhaps the most effective weapon that you can use to control others. Procrastination, another form of passive-aggressive anger, can also be used to control others. Constant depression may be a passive means of saying that you feel the world is no good, a cover for anger, or the result of anger. A well-ingrained pattern of forgetfulness, preoccupation, laziness, hypochondria, half-hearted efforts, blaming, verbal outbursts, gossiping, intimidation of others, and ruminating incessantly is a subtle expression of anger that prevents the honest communication of feelings.

Rules to guide the expression of anger into constructive methods would include:

One: Don't try to establish your superiority or claim special privileges because of your illness, when expressing anger.

Two: Deliberately select a constructive aim for expressing your anger. Doing this can turn the communication of that anger into a relational building tool.

Three: Be sensitive and aware of how responsive the person is that you wish to communicate with. Some things may be better left unsaid at a particular time because of the other persons' responsiveness. Since those who are intimately interwoven with your care may also be experiencing anger, establishing communication channels outside your immediate circle of family or friends may be helpful and even vital in blowing off excess anger. You can probably express your anger more honestly to someone who is not so caught up in your immediate situation. Let that person know that you are aware of "dumping" on him so he will know you are sensitive to his needs.

Four: Consider and understand, as best you can, the feelings and circumstances of the other person before expressing your anger. "Knowing when and how to express anger is the key. Just because it is sometimes correct to let it out doesn't mean that it is always correct. Sensitivity is the main trait that an angry person needs to hold onto" (Carter, p. 98).

Released Anger

Released anger is anger that is let go, and no longer needed. You can release anger only after you have learned how to recognize it, express it, and use it constructively to build relationships. Chronic illness can be such a source of anger about and toward so many things that there is danger of falling into a pattern of bitterness and loneliness as anger festers within.

In the process toward acceptance and mental wholeness, anger needs to be released, as well as expressed. When one emotion, such as anger, is bottled up, other emotions (like happiness, joy, and peace) also get "caught in the dam."

SUMMARY

Although anger will be experienced intermittently throughout life, a saturation point in the adjustment process may be reached when you are ready to move past the consuming anger that can accompany chronic illness. It is essential that the chronically ill learn to assertively express anger in a sensitive way and release it as part of moving through the grief process.

Relationships will suffer, and peace and laughter will be lost until you release your anger. "The people who remain constant slaves to anger are those who refuse to accept the responsibility for deciding their own destiny" (Carter, p. 99). You can be both "good" and "angry" at the same time. The way you handle anger ultimately reflects how you feel about yourself.

11

Depressed?

It's O.K. to be depressed!!! In fact, it would be *expected* of people coping with a chronic illness on a daily basis. It is estimated that even people who are healthy are depressed 40 percent of the time (Lanier, 1981) just from the stresses of daily living. Therefore, be kind and gentle with yourself.

Allow yourself to be depressed without criticism, feeling somehow that you don't measure up, or feeling you've failed. Depression is a message from your body and psyche back to you, trying to tell you something. Depression may be the result of expecting too much from yourself or from those around you.

Depression is a part of a *normal* cycle that *all* human beings go through. You can't expect yourself to cope effectively 100 percent of the time and to always have everything under control. Even the most experienced, polished juggler drops the balls at times, and has to stop to pick them up. Depression is normal and should be expected from time to time, on a recurring basis.

In the heat of the activity of dealing with a problem, an increase in health problems, or a crisis, emotions may be pushed to the back of the mind in order to be able to cope with and handle all the aspects of the situation effectively. As a solution is reached, health begins to improve, or the crisis passes, depression may hit like a herd of horses, or like thunder after the lightening.

You finally feel the full impact of the emotional toll that has been levied. It is after the crisis has passed and you are able to relax and look back, that you are most likely to be hit the hardest by depression.

If you find that depression is your constant frame of mind, then there may be a problem of greater severity that may require counseling or medication. Depression can feed on itself, producing more depression, if it is not recognized and dealt with. There needs to be an active recognition on your part to acknowledge depression and say to yourself or to someone else, "I am depressed." That's the start of dealing with it.

Once depression is acknowledged and labeled, you can actively try to do something to "head it off at the pass," so to speak. Basic here is the understanding that you alone are ultimately responsible for taking care of yourself. No one else can do it for you. Others only serve as encouragement or as guides.

You are the one who chooses how you are going to respond to every situation in life. Depression on an occasional basis is normal and expected; an "OK thing." You need a real good depression now and then—it's a kind of luxury. It's staying depressed all the time or on a more frequent basis that produces problems.

KEYS FOR DEALING
WITH DEPRESSION

Allow yourself to experience your depression to the fullest. You may need a break from being cheerful, brave, and having everything under control. Depression isn't all bad. It may give you a chance to "catch your second breath." You may have spent a lot of energy denying your anger and guilt, or your guilt about being angry. When you're on the bottom, there's only one way to go, and that's *up!*

In the cycle of adjustment, you may experience anger, denial, bargaining, depression, and acceptance. Depression is like hitting the wall of reality, experiencing the pain and tears, "letting it all hang out." It is the mechanism by which you are able to get on with life. "The person who doesn't experience depression is stuck in the denial stage and never comes to grips with himself" (Chyatte, 1979, p. 10). Don't run from it.

Key One: Allow yourself to experience the pain and reality where you are—at the bottom. Don't fight it or belittle yourself for being there. Know it's part of a process and need not last forever.

Depression can be a cover for more potent emotions you may not want to own up to, like anxiety, anger, or guilt. Depression indicates that there have been unacknowledged and unreleased thoughts producing emotions that have accumulated. Recognizing depression as a cover for other emotions may help you peek under the "covers" to see what's there.

Many times thoughts run about, bumping into each other and stimulating useless thought patterns, like a drunken monkey. Writing things down can bring a more logical sequence to thoughts and lead you out of confusion. When depressed, sitting down and making a list of things you may feel angry, guilty, or anxious about may help. It's like finding the loose end of a ball of yarn and unraveling it.

Key Two: Look below the surface to see what emotions are there. List what you may possibly feel angry, guilty, or anxious about.

Depression in chronic illness may come from many sources—the illness process itself, reaction to the illness, side effects from drugs, or reaction to life events or people. You need to get to know yourself well enough so that when depression hits, you can look back and perhaps tell where the depression was first kicked off. If you can't connect it with thoughts and emotions or with an event, it may well be due to the illness or drugs.

Key Three: Get to know yourself, your thoughts, and what triggers your depression.

"Depression and tears seem to be the mechanisms that restore the grieved to normalcy" (Chyatte, p. 10). Cry yourself a river, a lake, or an ocean. Tears are like a cleansing, healthy bath that washes away hurt and pain, giving vent to emotions. Strangely enough, a salty teardrop rolling off a cheek can carry the weight of many emotions. Preliminary findings of investigations into the chemistry of tears, by William Frey, Ph.D., show that tears contain enkephalin, a chemical produced by the body and thought to counteract pain.

If you find you can't cry, you may need to deliberately seek something out that will get the tears rolling. Somehow, crying alone may be more releasing. Crying with someone else can also be cleansing. The family that cries together may stay together.

Key Four: Don't be ashamed to cry. Allow yourself to shed some tears.

Research shows that exertion has beneficial effects in relieving depression. Circulation is stimulated to carry off wastes, and oxygen is carried to the cells. It seems that fatigue experienced upon waking in the morning may be more closely related to depression than physiological causes.

Sleep cycles may be disturbed with depression, creating more fatigue and depression. Exertion can tire the body, possibly producing better sleep. Fatigue can lead to depression, and depression can lead to fatigue.

Key Five: Some type of exertion on a regular basis (two or three times a week) may help break chronic depression/fatigue scenarios.

Research also shows that the cycles of night and day are reflected in bodily and emotional cycles. Depression seems to be more prevalent in the winter months when there is less light. Patients with pathological depression have shown improvement when exposed to longer cycles of bright light.

Key Six: Recognize that depression may be more prevalent during the winter months, when confined inside, or on rainy days, a widely accepted fact.

Nutrition has a definite effect on the emotions. What we eat is intimately interwoven with how we feel about ourselves. Depression tends to reduce appetite. Nutritional foods will be replaced by more appealing junk foods or candies. Good nutrition, however, is especially essential in times of stress.

Key Seven: Good nutrition and a well-balanced diet may slow or even help reverse a downward spiral of depression.

Identify special people in your life who can be a support and whom you can ask for help. That seems to be one of the most difficult things to do—admitting to people that you need them and their help. Share your situation with those people. They may not end up being the people who are closest to you. Just remember that you need more than one person to share your load with. A load shared is more easily shouldered.

Key Eight: Identify your key support people and let them know when you need them.

There will be certain dates or times of the year when depression is more prevalent. Try to mark in red on your calendar dates when you know you may be more susceptible to depression. Among these dates may be birthdays, anniversaries of good and bad times, and holidays. All are potent with emotions.

Key Nine: Deliberately plan an activity or treat that you really enjoy for those days when you are most prone to depression.

With the onset of illness, a very active life may come to a standstill. Idleness may replace activity, boredom may drown vitality, and an all-consuming preoccupation with the self may push aside interest in life. These occurrences may create a fertile climate for depression. If part of getting sick is focusing on the self, then part of getting well is focusing *outside* the self.

Key Ten: Establish schedules, write down things you need to do, and check them off when done. Stay involved with others, whether by mail, phone, newspapers, or television.

When you are depressed, you normally focus on the internal functioning of your body. Any symptom, ache, or pain may become magnified and intensified beyond its realistic significance. Pain and other bodily complaints can mask depression, since all concern and attention may be focused on the physical problem. Unhappiness inherent in depression can be concealed or avoided by shifting attention to your pain or feeling bad. When depressed, pain can be generated from emotional as well as physical sources.

Key Eleven: When experiencing increased pain and/or depression, try to realistically fathom which is which by recognizing that they sometimes go hand in hand. Try to treat the problem from both directions, as pain and/or depression, and see which approach works best. Both entities can cause and make the other worse.

SUMMARY

Being depressed is no fun, but it seems to be a fact of life. Rather than wallowing in it when it comes, you can educate yourself about it and use it as a constructive mechanism for growth, insight, breaking down walls and creating doors, and developing a sensitivity for life and for those around you also shouldering burdens.

It may take some breaking down in order to put the pieces back together in a healthier fashion. Experiencing the rain can make the sunshine seem that much brighter. Depression can be visualized as valleys of life that can teach you how to build bridges over troubled waters.

12

Acceptance!?

Some people think of acceptance of a chronic illness as either complete capitulation or total vigilance, but actually it is neither. Acceptance is, in reality, an integral part of life. You accept a gift, a compliment, a job offer, someone's love, a challenge. To accept is defined as "to receive or take in, hold, or contain." Another definition refers to acceptance as "being done willingly or gladly." Acceptance of a chronic illness, however, would be done out of necessity, not willingly or gladly.

"Capitulation refers to the person who, under the sentence of ill health, goes to pieces and essentially renounces the idea of remaining himself. To accept means to keep a firm grip on yourself and to work toward safeguarding your integrity. Acceptance implies a refusal to be condemned or to give up and become a useless person in the face of diminishing health. There is an element of non-acceptance in this kind of acceptance" (Werner–Beland, 1980, p. 1976).

There are some hallmarks of acceptance that will be evident to the chronically ill and those around them. Included among these are:

1. *It is no longer necessary to focus on the illness or one's self.* For a while this is necessary, but there comes a time when the illness becomes only a part of your life and not its main focus. "Sometimes it is tempting to let that illness become an idol—the most important aspect in your life becomes your God" (Cox-Gedmark, 1980, p. 113).

2. A corollary to this is that *you begin to see the needs of others again.* "Many troubled people beome highly egocentric in the sense that they can view their problem and situation only from their own

perspective" (Kanfer-Goldstein, 1980, pp. 68-69). You may feel you are unique and that no one's problems can equal yours.

3. *The illness blends in as only a part of your total identity,* such that everyone doesn't *have* to know about it.

4. On the other hand, *you shouldn't have to go to great lengths to hide the illness,* either. Acceptance requires that a person absorb it within his psychological outlook in such a way that it is no longer a painful fact that must be concealed. Trying to forget is the best way of remembering (Wright, 1960, p. 23).

5. *Illness' effects become contained so they do not affect all situations in life.*

6. *Being able to identify with people who have similar conditions shows acknowledgement of changes seen in the self.*

7. "To accept . . . by no means implies an all-absorbing interest in illness-connected problems. Too much preoccupation may be as much a sign of maladjustment as ostensibly too little" (Wright, p. 47). *A well-rounded life is preferable with many interests,* possibly old interests as well as new ones.

8. *Acceptance must be on an intellectual and emotional level.* Over-intellectualization may be a form of denial. There must also be gut-level emotional grieving. Intellectual acceptance may lead the way to emotional acceptance.

9. *Feelings of bitterness, defensiveness, and anger are released* when you no longer see yourself as a victim but as a participant, and assume responsibility for yourself.

10. *Fears become more realistic* instead of a generalized, consuming anxiety.

11. *Accept yourself, shed self-pity, and become comfortable with yourself and those around you.*

12. *Accept the reality of your limitations and learn to ask for help in an assertive way, not aggressively, whimpering, or complaining, but bargaining your limitations.*

13. *Try to see humor in your situation and learn to laugh and play again.*

14. *Set new goals when old ones are no longer realistic.*

15. *Reaching acceptance seems to link with the return of hope.* "The attitudes of acceptance, patience, and ultimately hope, are difficult to maintain . . ." (Werner-Beland, p. 178).

16. *See yourself as being no different from others,* only an "average Joe" handling your problems as well as possible—no martyr, saint, or anyone special.
17. *Be able to identify with the similarities of others* and not just with your differences.
18. *See yourself as a person of value as you are right now.*
19. *Learn to listen to, understand, and trust yourself.*

"A person can react in three different ways to a chronic illness. The first is to give up. The second is to fight the diagnosis continually, which leads to despair because you get nowhere. The third road is to get active in your own behalf and take responsibility for your well-being and your goals for the future." (Cox-Gedmark, p. 55).

SUMMARY

Acceptance is like a see-saw. Part of you wants to get on with life as it is now and another part wants to stay with the loss. It takes a lot of time, patience, love, determination, and understanding. Acceptance is a day-by-day experience, as things are continually changing. Having reached these hallmarks once (there are others as well) gives promise that you can continue to capitalize on them. Although you never fully reach acceptance once and for all, it's only through the doors of ongoing acceptance of life in the "now" that you can discover peace and joy.

13

"Diagnostic Crazies"

"Listen, Doc, what's going on? I have all these aches and pains. I feel lousy all the time. I'm tired, grouchy, and just can't seem to function like I used to. I push and try but I just can't seem to get my act together."

"I feel so angry and guilty. My husband, family, and friends can't understand why I'm acting so strangely. Neither can I. Friends are getting tired of asking how I'm doing. When they ask what's wrong, I don't know what to tell them anymore."

"My boss thinks I'm dragging my feet and has made hints about his dissatisfaction with my performance. I should be in line for a promotion and raise about now, but instead, I'm afraid he may fire me if I don't straighten up and get back to 'normal.' I feel like I'm getting to be a chronic complainer and I was never that way before now. I used to be such a positive, active person. I feel like I'm becoming a different person!"

"I don't know how much longer all these people are going to have patience with me without some answers as to what's going on. Please tell me what's wrong with me so I can take some medicine and get on with my life! You've run so many tests. I don't want anything to be wrong with me, but I know there has to be or I wouldn't be feeling as bad as I do. Please, tell me what I have . . . now!!"

THE SETTING

Sitting in the same room, facing this distraught person (maybe you), is a physician who has devoted his life to a career in medicine, sometimes at great financial and personal sacrifice. He uses all his knowledge and experience to put the pieces of the puzzle (your symptoms or illness) together and come up with a correct diagnosis.

In response to your insistent, impassioned pleas, the physician may be tempted to hastily put a diagnosis on your chart, just to have the matter settled and get you out of his hair. It takes much greater honesty to say, "No, I don't know exactly what is going on with you."

You have your own beliefs, attitudes, and conceptions about illness, together with all kinds of good and bad prejudices about doctors (Benet, 1979, p. 26). Some of these ideas may be generated from the myth concerning the power of our modern technology and medicine and the perception of the physician as "God-like."

You may be sitting there thinking simplistically that any condition can be easily diagnosed, or unrealistically thinking that there is a cure or pill for your every ache and pain. Just watching TV for an hour or so will reinforce this belief. Rather than viewing medicine as an "imperfect, fallible science," you may view it as a "perfect, infallible science." It isn't!!

On the other hand, the physician may be sitting there, knowing that medicine is an imperfect science with many limitations, even when doing its best. Many conditions, such as neuromuscular abnormalities, connective tissue/immune complex illnesses and others, can be very difficult to diagnose. Diagnosing such conditions may require time, meticulous lab work-ups, thorough medical histories, and sometimes trials on medication. Even with the diagnosis, there may be no cure or treatment with easy answers, but only trial–and–error to see what helps.

THE CHARACTERS

Here you have two people approaching diagnosis from two different viewpoints; one very personal, and one professional as well as personal. You may have reached the point of frustration bordering on becoming irrational, with diagnosis becoming an obsession.

You both want answers. But, more than likely, when the answers and diagnosis you have been waiting for arrive, they aren't what you wanted to hear, although at first there may be a great deal of relief to finally have a diagnosis. You may feel that your whole being and credibility are "on the line."

The physician is probably there for many reasons—to make a living, to practice his learned profession, to help people. He wants to be correct in his diagnosis and may be just as frustrated as you are, for different reasons. A professional cool must be maintained so that the situation can be viewed with clinical objectivity. To some degree, the physician's being and credibility may also be "on the line."

RESULTS OF A DIAGNOSIS

For the physician, a correct diagnosis may represent a validation of his professional expertise, providing positive strokes for the "ol' ego," as well as the personal gratification of helping another human being. The diagnosis provides a starting point for the ongoing treatment and monitoring of the patient.

Diagnosing a disease allows a physician to get on with things. Treatment and medications can be prescribed, help offered, and advice given. Your doctor can monitor your condition as you hopefully see steady improvement. Some doctors may be more adept at diagnosis, while others may be better attuned to treatment.

A number of things may occur as you are diagnosed. You take on a new identity with that diagnosis. By this point, you may have had serious doubts about your sanity. Doubts of this nature may have been voiced by a physician or two along the way, as well as by family or friends.

Up to this point, your experience of your internal reality, being sick, may not have been verified or validated in your external reality. When the experience of the outside world and the inside world don't correlate, you have a unique type of insanity, all by itself. Diagnosis may bring a meshing of the two. Then, again, your worst fears may be realized, putting your sanity to yet another test.

Result One: With a diagnosis, your perceptions of your inner reality are validated in your external world. At the same time, the diagnosis that you feared and may not be quite ready to accept is validated. It has been put into words, and typed in bold print on both your chart and your life.

It is difficult to face the unknown, with all its uncertainties generating anxiety and fear. Knowing what you're dealing with and putting a label on its dispels some of the unknowns, possibly giving a feeling of control. At the same time, a diagnosis may generate another whole list of unknowns. Absolute answers, easy solutions, and guarantees are not to be had in this life.

Result Two: Diagnosis can dispel some of the unknowns and create others. With or without a diagnosis, there will be some degree of anxiety and fear related to the unknowns and uncertainties in life. There may not be answers to every question.

Putting a diagnosis of a disease on an illness does, at least, condense what you are experiencing into a more manageable form of communication. A single word or grouping of words can replace the long list of complaints used previously to explain what is wrong with you. Your own subjective experience may be questioned, but an objective label given by a physician is an undeniable, authentic description that most people don't question.

A diagnosis of a recognized disease is essential when trying to communicate your needs officially to, for example, an employer, insurance companies, or disability reviews. Vague complaints and symptoms just don't cut it in this arena. At this time, a diagnosis can become a label that allows people to put you in a box. They can't see beyond that label to get to know you. A diagnosis of a medically and publically recognized disease can confine as well as liberate you.

Result Three: A diagnosis can be a useful communication tool in many situations, but it can also be used by others to confine you to that label, never bothering to get to know the rest of you.

An official diagnostic decree uttered by a physician puts what you are experiencing into definite descriptive terms. This decree "allows you" to feel bad, to own what you are experiencing as illness. It thereby gives you permission to take care of yourself and not try so hard to appear "normal."

You can now give in to your fatigue or pain and do something about it, rather than bravely push on and on. At the same time, you may have to sit down and take a long, hard look at the way you are going about your life, making some drastic, unwanted changes in lifestyle.

Result Four: A diagnosis may give you permission to take care of yourself, but it may also be a mandate that brings about many drastic, unwanted changes in the way you live and how you view yourself.

The ultimate results of a diagnosis would hopefully be treatment, with relief of symptoms and an improved lifestyle. That dream might be only partially true. Sometimes, you may look forward to a diagnosis as the "pot of gold at the end of the rainbow," the proof that you were right, the answer to all your questions and the solution to all problems.

As with the doctor, the diagnosis only serves as a sober beginning, not the end of a quest. Some questions may not be answered, some problems aren't going to go away and may have to be lived with, and more problems than solutions may be created. A diagnosis can be a short-lived victory but it can give guidance and clarification to what has been happening to you. It is much easier to live with some unknowns than with all unknowns.

Result Five: A diagnosis is just the beginning of a journey. It opens the door to perhaps a few new problems, but may close the door on some old ones.

SUMMARY

I know there have been times in my own journey with chronic illness when, out of frustration, I might have "sold my soul" for a diagnosis to give answers to the "why's" of my body's limitations—the "diagnostic crazies!!!" Along the road of chronic illness, I've found this to happen on a recurring basis.

I would construct my own rationale and put myself through frantic self-examination while asking for every diagnostic test in the book. Ultimately, when nothing could be found "diagnostically" to explain what I was experiencing, I would have to trust my own inner experience and reality, not doubt myself or become impatient or angry with my physician, acknowledge and live within my body's definition of its limitations, and not make a diagnosis my main focus.

As smart as the physician is and as wonderful as all the modern diagnostic procedures are, just because he can't find diagnostic proof to substantiate or support what you are experiencing doesn't mean that it isn't there and you aren't experiencing it.

The important thing is to learn to trust yourself while, at the same time, keeping an open mind to those around you, listening to your body, and telling your physician what it says, accepting it with all its weird unexplained symptoms. Trust that the answers will be down the road somewhere if they are important enough. The essential thing is to learn to *live* within those limitations and symptoms in an uncritical way, whether they are defined or sanctioned medically, with a diagnosis or not!

PART III

Looking at the Medical Side of Chronic Illness

14

"What's Up, Doc?"

"Oops! I forgot to ask my doctor about that medicine. By golly, I failed to tell him about my rash! My mind gets so boggled and I get so tongue-tied at doctor's visits! I can't remember when something started, or how!" Does this sound familiar, or ever happen to you?

When first being diagnosed with a chronic illness, I would come away from my doctor's appointments totally frustrated. There would be so much happening between visits that I would want to get a reading or an impression of from my doctor.

Without fail, I would forget something or go completely blank in the emotionally–heightened atmosphere of a doctor's visit. This would result in frustration and unresolved anxiety. Over the years I began developing a system that I feel has helped me communicate with my doctor, who has most graciously adapted to this idiosyncracy of mine.

Between visits, I keep a running diary of occurrences that I feel my doctor should be aware of. Using a "month-at-a-glance" calendar may be a good way to keep up with this, watch for patterns, and put together cause –and–effect for problems. I also jot down questions that might come to mind. By writing them down, I don't have to try to remember each item, and I can get it off my mind. This frees me for involvement in other things. A day or so before the visit, I go over my list of questions and problems.

I scratch off some things that might have been resolved on their own and not have proven to be significant, or I might add others. Some items might not be of great concern or significance in terms of altering treatment, but might give the doctor a picture of ongoing or declining disease activity. Other items might be of greater concern and significance.

On my updated list, I include physical symptoms, emotional state (if having problems), appointments with other doctors, what other doctors have said at visits with me, information about work status or current involvements, billing problems—anything that might give a complete picture of what is going on with me.

I type or write my update list and questions as neatly as possible, making a carbon copy. I include the date, the doctor's name, my updated list, and then my questions and present concerns. It is easier to carefully word what I want to say rather than try to verbalize it. This is particularly helpful when seeing several doctors. You have a way of checking what you have mentioned to which doctor, and when.

At my visit, I give my doctor a copy of my updated list, questions, and present concerns to keep. This allows him to scan what I have put down, commenting on items he feels are significant and need follow-up, and passing over less important items. If he doesn't pick up on something I'm concerned about or particularly want a reading on, I reinforce it verbally.

Not having to discuss each item leaves more time to discuss the most important points. Information that might have been forgotten or not clearly communicated is transmitted. I keep my carbons, write information about tests, their results, answers to questions, and file them.

This system has come to serve as a diary that gives me feedback concerning my symptoms as correlated with lab results, and illness fluctuations as related to other parts of my life. It also helps me observe disease activity and patterns in relation to seasonal changes and activities.

In addition to serving as my personal diary, it can also serve as a source of valuable documentation if needed for insurance or disability purposes. It is difficult to rely just on memory for certain dates or events. Using this approach has met many of my needs.

I still forget things and end up calling back or writing to my doctor! Even so, I usually feel we've covered a lot of ground during a visit. From my doctor's response I can pick up on which things to just add to the "live with it" list while keeping an eye on them as an indication of disease activity, and which things might need more attention with additional follow-up.

SUMMARY

You may want to try this process, including your own variations and ideas. It may work for you and your doctor and it may not. Give it a try! The intent is for you to be able to establish an agenda that is important to you during your visit with your doctor so that you feel you have communicated well in a limited time frame. There can be no doctor/patient partnership without adequate communication between the two partners. You need to carry your part of this partnership.

15

Hospitalizations

Hospitalizations will occur from time to time when living with a chronic illness. Time in the hospital may be needed during acute exacerbations of the chronic illness, when other illnesses are added in, for re-evaluations or diagnostic work-up, for corrective surgery due to degenerative changes. Whatever the reason, going into the hospital isn't anticipated with great joy.

A period of hospitalization may send signals to those people around you of a close or casual nature. Awareness of your illness-related problems may increase. Some of these problems may have been present all along but ignored by many. This time of increased awareness and attention, with the forces rallying to bring in meals and help out, may be particularly embarrassing for children or teenagers as well as for you and the whole family.

Procedures that need to be endured during a hospital stay may be even more difficult to cope with than the illness itself. Here are some tips that may help you to make it through a hospital stay:

1. *"NPO" (Nothing by Mouth)* for patients with a dry mouth, Sjögren's Syndrome, presents special problems:
    *   rinse mouth out with mouthwash or brush teeth, being careful not to swallow
    *   suck a slightly damp washrag, letting dry mucous membranes absorb the moisture
    *   keep lips moistened with lip balm
    *   drink plenty of fluids right up to the time for "NPO" to begin
    *   ask for a vaporizer.

2. Put alcohol on raw elbows to dry them out, making them tougher (the sheets won't rub as much this way).

3. To ease nausea:
   • eat small, frequent meals
   • try deep abdominal breathing
   • chew on or suck on ice chips
   • drink carbonated beverages or hot tea
   • apply a cold compress to forehead
   • eat dry toast or crackers.

4. Bring extra pillows from home to help position painful joints. When lying on side, a pillow between the knees can prevent hip rotation. Use a pillow to support arm and shoulder.

5. Change bed position to help alleviate back discomfort with sciatic pain, sore joints, or difficulty breathing when lying flat—raise the head up over half way with knee gatch elevated.

6. Cheese crackers, if permitted in diet, help take away bad taste of medications.

7. Use cotton balls or ear plugs to shut out hospital or roommate's noises so you can sleep.

8. Dry heat in hospital dries out sinuses—vaporizer provides moisture and its quiet noise helps to drown out other noises.

9. When pain or discomfort is intense, mental imagery of beautiful scenery or pleasant memories can help to make it more bearable.

10. Isometric exercises (tightening and relaxing muscle groups), wiggling toes, flexing muscles, and deep-breathing exercises (even while confined to bed) can help promote relaxation and increase circulation.

11. Some procedures require lying still in uncomfortable positions for long periods of time. Try:
    • focusing on points in room to provide a diversion
    • wiggling toes or any part of the body in a rotating manner.

12. Take extra blankets and a pair of socks to cover cold hands and feet that accompany Raynaud's phenomenon (contraction of vessels in hands and feet) in possibly cool hospital temperatures. Cold hands and feet may be a problem for you even without Raynaud's.

Going into the hospital may bolster your credibility of being sick with family, friends, health care professionals or insurance providers. It's difficult for most people to realize that illness can be experienced on an ongoing daily basis while remaining functional and even cheerful. "If you are able to be up and about, surely what you're experiencing isn't serious or significant . . ." not so!

SUMMARY

You and your family's emotional, physical, and financial resources may be drained as hospitalizations turn family routines, schedules, and budgets into chaos. All may be strained to meet the increased demands. Visits or phone calls from friends and family may be inappropriate, adding to the strain rather than helping. You need to be honest with your supportive community, telling them what you and your family do and don't need to help you through this difficult time.

16

Medical Word Games

Words have no meaning except in the way you interpret and respond to them from your own experience. The same words may hold different meaning for you as your life unfolds and you experience their reality from different angles.

At one point, a word may be experienced with fear and depression. At another point, the reaction to the same word may be nonchalant or blasé. It is only when your life translates a word into a living definition and experience that you fully understand its meaning. Until that time, it remains just a word. Many descriptive words may be used medically to classify, categorize, or provide a tool for communication about an illness for medical personnel. These words, learned in training, may hold no meaning for them, personally.

MILD / SEVERE

In medical jargon, an illness may be categorized as "mild" or "severe." To the person living with the illness, there is nothing "mild" about it. Being told you have a "mild" case of anything may be received with mixed emotions, or as a slap in the face.

A condition that creates havoc with your lifestyle, pain, confusion, changed relationships and self-image, or fatigue, relates to nothing of a "mild" nature. The classification of "mild" seems to indicate that things should be "almost normal," or that it shouldn't be so bad. That's not always the case. For example, fatigue, sore muscles and joints may be more limiting than decreased kidney functioning.

In the medical sense, the word "mild" implies that the condition is not "life-threatening" or has no serious long-term implications. This gives no picture of your subjective experiences. You may find yourself thinking, "If this is *mild*, I'd hate to see what *severe* is!" Even though a "mild" condition may not result in death, you may *feel* like "death warmed over."

When considering a condition such as systemic lupus erythematosus (*SLE*, an autoimmune collagen vascular disease), the patient with "mild" disease activity may experience fever, arthritis, inflammation of the lung and / or heart lining with small collections of fluid around either, fatigue, rash. In the way of thinking of the general public, there is nothing "mild" about any such symptoms. None of these complaints could be considered "normal," and anything outside the realm of "normal" is not "mild."

"Severe," in medical terms, indicates a condition that may be "life-threatening" or has serious long-term implications. Strange as it may seem, the person with "severe" disease activity may not feel as awful or be as incapacitated over long periods of time as the person with ongoing "mild" problems. Although "mild" disease isn't "life-threatening," it can be "life-stifling."

Since the "severe" situation is so potentially dangerous, with the "big gun" drugs or treatments aimed at it, relief may be seen on the horizon. On the other hand, many symptoms may have to be endured with "mild" disease, since the risks of upping the potentially more toxic drugs are not warranted. You don't shoot a mosquito with a shotgun and take your foot off with it. One of the watchwords of the medical profession is "Do no harm."

Large amounts of attention and empathy may be heaped on "severe" cases, as should be. "Mild" cases may find treatment delivered in a more nonchalant manner. Interest of friends and family may come and go. Necessary, expensive lab tests may be run on a regular basis over and over as a matter of routine monitoring with no subsequent change in treatment or condition. Necessary drug bills may sap the budget without any expectation that you're going to feel "good" as a result.

NORMAL / ABNORMAL

"Abnormal" lab work or symptoms may produce a real flurry of concern and activity for a time after the initial diagnosis. As the months and years go by and disease activity establishes a pattern, the very same lab results may be accompanied with congratulations rather than concern. You are slowly establishing what is "significantly abnormal" for you or what is your "normal abnormal" and "abnormal abnormal" in terms of lab work and symptoms.

At one point, anything "abnormal" would have been "significant." You slowly learn to live within different parameters, accept trade-offs, and incorporate "mild" symptoms into your life, even though their consequences in terms of your altered way of living may not be "mild."

ACUTE / CHRONIC

Some other medical terms used to categorize illness are "acute" and "chronic sub-acute." "Acute," although there is nothing "cute" about it, is defined medically as a condition having "severe" symptoms and an expected short course.

The general public is more knowledgeable about this type of illness. You either improve and get well, or get worse, become terminal, and die. The adrenaline pumps, quick solutions are aggressively sought and applied, and results are or aren't evident within a short time. There is an end in sight.

"Chronic sub-acute" implies a condition that may persist for a long time, showing little change or progressing slowly over a long period of time. As opposed to "acute" or "terminal" illness, the pace of dealing with "chronic" illness must be slower and more methodical in order to prevent "burn-out."

Strength and coping abilities may have to stretch out over long periods of time, with many bumps in the road throughout life. You may not get completely well or die, but must learn to live with fluctuations in the ongoing illness. Your lifestyle may have to change in many ways, continuing to alter through the years.

"Chronic sub-acute" illness is the long-distance marathon that requires endurance, determination not to give up, bulldog tenacity, and ability to "stick-to-it" in order to "go the distance." Your pace needs to be well timed and flexible. "Acute" illness, in comparison, is the sprint.

"Acute" episodes or flares can be interspersed within a "chronic sub-acute" illness. The balancing game of what approach to take may get tangled between the sprints and marathon. Both approaches may have to be used at the same time—a real juggling act. These sprints may break your pace and sap your energy for the long-distance marathon.

PROGRESSIVE / PHASIC

"Progressive" and "phasic" are two more terms used in the medical community. "Progressive" carries the connotation of continuous spreading or increasing severity, with a downhill course potentially leading to death or a gloomy outcome.

"Phasic" describes a come-and-go type of activity exhibited by illnesses such as systemic lupus erythematosus (SLE), rheumatoid arthritis (RA), and multiple sclerosis (MS). A phasic illness involves erratic, unpredictable, up-and-down, back-and-forth motion with no clear-cut course of illness, recovery, and / or prognosis. When you think about it, life itself is "phasically progressive."

DISEASE / ILLNESS

Now, here's a tricky one that really "splits hairs." Illness and disease are not the same thing. "Any set of symptoms (the illness) can be ascribed to one of a finite number of possible anatomic or physiologic derangements (the disease)" (Hadler, 1982, p. 667). For instance, a sore throat or joint, or low back pain, are symptoms of an illness. They are not a disease in and of themselves.

"The quest for the disease, the cause of each patient's illness, is the diagnostician's banner and the focus of therapy" (Hadler, p. 667). Erroneously, many people feel that if a disease is identified, the illness is predictable. The diagnosis of a disease seems to put fragmented symptoms of an illness together into a completed puzzle, but in no way offer any magic control or treatment.

A chronic illness implies ongoing sets of symptoms and health problems that can be linked together as expressions of an underlying disease produced by anatomic or physiologic derangements. Unrelated health events may be related by way of a disease—a family of symptoms.

Your illness symptoms may be sore joints, fatigue, fever, weakness, muscle aches, or pains, but your disease may be multiple sclerosis (MS), heart disease, diabetes, systemic lupus erythematosus (SLE), rheumatoid arthritis (RA), or cancer. Confusing?

CURABLE / INCURABLE

A cure may be defined as the eradication of a disease, the course of treatment to restore health, the restoration of health, recovery from a disease, healing, or a remedy. The slate is wiped clean of symptoms of illness produced by a disease. Sometimes, time requirements for the absence of symptoms or problems are necessary before a condition can be considered cured, such as cancer.

Incurable may be defined as not susceptible or capable of being cured, not susceptible to modification, or a person with a disease that cannot be cured. Incurable also implies that no cause has been discovered for the disease. You need to know what's broken and why before you can fix it. Similarly, the cause of a disease must be determined before a cure can be found.

Chronic illness is incurable and usually the symptoms of the illness produced by a disease are treated rather than the disease itself. The slate can't be wiped clean, but is kept as usable as possible. The causes of more and more diseases are being pinpointed, providing prevention or cure (for example, tuberculosis, smallpox, polio, and cancer), offering hope and encouragement for all. Research progress in one area may open doors to advances in other medical areas.

SUMMARY

Words shouldn't control you or your reactions, but should serve as a means of expression and a communication tool to tell others about your experience of life. Unfamiliar words may produce fear, anxiety, and panic. You need to live those words and educate yourself about what they mean and say to you in order to evolve your own personal definition.

As a nurse, I used all of these terms casually, but learning to live with them and to integrate them into my living as they personally apply to me has been a whole different matter. Words can be used as a game to avoid reality, or they can be used to give meaning, understanding, clarity, and definition to your world.

17

New Thoughts on Pain

Is pain merely a connection of pathways of nerves from the source of the pain to the brain and back? Can there be another learned social component to pain that affects the way you experience, perceive, and handle it?

If pain involves a learned social component, can approaches to pain other than conventional medication and surgery be of help in handling it? Can the internal resources of your mind be utilized to deal with pain? Why do some people have high pain tolerance and others low pain tolerance?

These questions are the seeds of thought that Dr. Nathaniel H. Hollister raises. Dr. Hollister is a neurosurgeon with a great deal of experience in working with people in pain. His many years of encounter have brought him to pose such questions and to try to develop new approaches in helping people cope with *real, genuine pain*, not imagined pain or pain that is "just in the head."

In order to try these new approaches out, Dr. Hollister stresses that you must allow your belief system to incorporate a broader concept of pain than merely the nerve connections to and from the brain. You need to weigh and consider other factors carefully and with an open mind.

Pain is a perceptual experience. That is, you first become aware of it through one of your senses, and then translate it into something meaningful. The quality and intensity of your pain is influenced by your unique past experience, by the meaning you assign to the cause of pain, and by your state of mind at the moment the pain is experienced.

Much pain behavior is learned in the family unit and culture in which you were raised. Pain is an individual, pervasive experience. Pain behaviors learned in the family unit are then tried out, reinforced or extinguished, maintained or adapted by your culture.

Studies of different cultural groups have shown varied responses to pain. Patients of Italian origin seemed mainly concerned with the immediate sensations of pain, welcomed relief provided by pain medication, and ceased to worry when the pain was gone. Jewish patients tended to focus mainly on what the pain meant to their general health and resisted pain medication. However, they remained worried when the pain was gone. Both groups felt free to talk and complain about their pain (Shontz, 1975, p. 234).

Third generation Americans worried about the implications of their pain, tried to be "good" patients, stoically withdrew while bearing pain, tried to resist any emotional response, and seemed optimistic about their future, due to trust in medical science. As such, they did not dwell on their pain (Shontz, p. 234).

Response to pain seems more favorable when the pain is predictable and within the person's control. Patients educated preoperatively about what will happen postoperatively require less pain medication and recover more quickly after surgery than those not educated. Greater pain is experienced when the circumstances surrounding the cause of your pain are ambiguous and complex. Fear and anxiety fan the flames of pain, especially if the pain is interpreted as being from a life-threatening source.

When your pain is associated with a beneficial state of affairs, such as in childbirth or winning a game, it is not accompanied by anxiety. Suffering is then minimized. There are many stories of athletes with major injuries finishing a game or an event, only to collapse in pain afterwards.

It has been found that patients who communicate openly with their physicians require less pain medication. "Possibly, the relief that many patients experience through talking about their conditions stems from the reduction of psychological tension rather than reduction of physical pain as such" (Shontz, p. 90)

Pain seems to be more intense when you are alone, at night, or when you have no source of help or nothing to take your mind off it. Pain gets worse when the doctor is unavailable, like at night or during weekends, and when there is reduced outside stimulation to divert attention from the pain. Pain may astonishingly improve while on the way to see the doctor.

Pain tolerance is reduced with high anxiety, depression, highly concentrating on bodily functions, an introverted personality, and focusing on the internal stimuli from your body so that pain is perceived as more intense and poorly tolerated. Pain tolerance is increased with low anxiety, minimal concentration on your bodily functions, an extroverted personality, and focusing on external stimuli.

Some people tend to augment their own pain or intensify it and others, to reduce the pain and its effects. Two keys seem to be dealing with anxiety and staying in touch with stimuli from the outside world. Anxiety may be reduced with knowing what the pain means and providing a means of relief, whether it involves heat, traction, bracing, mechanical devices, cold, massage, relaxation techniques, imagery, pain medication, exercise, diversion, family and cultural dynamics, or your own unique personality and belief system.

Chronic pain lends itself more readily to adopting learned behaviors that become a form of communication to those around us than does acute, short-lived pain. The circumstances and responses of people around you can either reinforce your pain behavior through secondary gains such as increased attention and reducing anxiety and responsibility, or negate pain behaviors.

In a study of families dealing with chronic pain, it was found that the spouse's coping mechanisms revealed a noticeable lack of resources, such as a support system found in religious faith; talking with other family members, doctors, or others; and seeking information about the source, meaning, or ways of relieving the chronic pain (Rowat, 1983, p. 213). It was also found that spouses who were highly stressed from other sources had the least resources to cope with the situation. Therefore, they handled the situation in a more stressful manner for all concerned.

Roles that spouses assumed in coping with chronic pain varied from the protector-advocate, to the instructor-admonisher, to the avoider-ignorer (Rowat, p. 168). The protector role, involving many maneuvers on behalf of the spouse to insulate the partner in chronic pain, was found to be the most depleting of the roles (p. 190). "If one believes his coping resources are depleted then he may perceive transactions as threatening where they otherwise would not be" (p. 218). A combining or shifting among all the roles may be the most realistic approach.

Pain may be rewarded and reinforced by health care professionals when they give you increased amounts of attention, and pain medication on a PRN (as needed) schedule rather than a regular schedule. They may encourage you to rest at the first sign of pain rather than before it appears. One of the first questions that may be asked by physicians and friends alike is, "Are you in pain?" It's a definite attention-getting device!

Dr. Hollister's approach stresses the use of interpersonal communication technology, neurolinguistic programming, to control painful conditions. Pain is a message from the body that is, in turn, interpreted and communicated both verbally and / or nonverbally.

Many other things not mentioned here affect what pain means to the individual, how it is experienced, and what is done with it. Pain behaviors, such as limping, wincing, and sighing, are usually reduced when you are alone, and exaggerated when significant others are present. The more you learn about it, the more complex the topic of pain becomes.

SUMMARY

There's a lot to learn about pain in general and how you experience your own pain. The topic isn't as simple as you might think. There are resources in your area that can be used to further explore this topic. Since pain can set up a stress cycle that may stimulate, prolong, and intensify chronic illness activity, it behooves you to learn all you can about the topic and how it applies to you individually.

PART IV

Looking at the Personal Side of Chronic Illness

18

Emotional Maintenance

Everything in this life is subject to "wear and tear." Any appliance, car, watch, piece of equipment, or house you buy comes with a guarantee or maintenance contract to cover the posibility of malfunction or breakdown. You take your car for regular maintenance checks to keep it in top working condition.

Adequate rest, a well-balanced diet, and exercise are all forms of maintenance work in caring for your body. You are encouraged to get a physical check-up, pap smear, and dental exam, among other tests, at regular intervals.

In contrast, you seldom think of maintenance as involving the emotions. Modern-day science and medicine recognize that stress has an impact on both your emotions and your body. You can't treat or ignore one without treating or ignoring aspects of the other.

It has been found that no direct correlation can be drawn from a particular personality type to a specific illness, or vice–versa, but illness and the emotions are definitely interrelated and affect each other. There is indeed a mind/body connection.

In the 1960's, there was emphasis on the relationship between major life events (divorce, death, job change, marriage, promotion, pregnancy) and physical condition within the next year or two. Different major life events were given a numerical value based on their estimated impact as stressors. There seemed to be a cumulative effect in that, the more life changes present in a year's span, the greater the likelihood of illness later on.

Emphasis has recently shifted to focus on the stress produced by everyday hassles. "Daily hassles seem to be more closely linked to and may have a greater effect on your moods and on your health than the major misfortunes. Major life events, in addition to their obvious or immediate impact, can create continuing hassles—a kind of 'ripple effect' " (Lazarus, 1981, p. 60-61). Being diagnosed with a chronic illness is a major life event that has great impact, translating into many everyday hassles.

Stress tends to accumulate over time, resulting in a stress spiral. When you are already stressed, a neutral event that you ordinarily might not respond to sends your stress level even higher. With the next stress, you start out at a higher level, going even higher. Your chances of recovery from the stress arousal spiral diminish with each succeeding stress. Failure to recover from stress arousal may lead to problems.

You need to build something into your daily life that promotes recovery from stress. What you do to build stress recovery into your life depends on how you respond to stress. Generally, people handle stress either cognitively/mentally, somatically/physically, or a combination of the two.

In the mental response, the person becomes fixated on the stress or problem, ruminating on it continually—going over it in his mind in a compulsive way. The physical response is exhibited by muscle tenseness, sweating, increased blood pressure, pulse, and respirations which can be measured by biofeedback techniques.

In the mental response, the recovery approach would be aimed at breaking the thought pattern or taking the mind off the stress. In the physical response, the recovery approach would use physical change to break or release body tension. Below is a grid showing different response combinations and examples of stress recovery approaches.

SUMMARY

Hans Selye, the "Father" of the study of stress, feels that we all have a limited amount of adaptation energy to handle stress. When your adaptation energy is gone, it's gone, and you break down physically, emotionally, or both. You may have already tried some of the approaches mentioned, as well as others. You may have found some that worked and

STRESS RECOVERY APPROACHES

Physical: High Mental: Low		Physical: High Mental: High	
Aerobics	Jogging	Auto-hypnosis	Primal scream
Bicycling	Massage	Biofeedback	Sex
Dance	Sex	Martial arts	Video games
Deep breath- ing/isometrics	Swimming Walking	Meditation	Yoga
Hot tub			
Physical: Low Mental: Low		Physical: Low Mental: High	
		Counselling	Reading
Any of the items listed		Cultural events	Rubik's cube
		Friends	Sewing
		Journaling	Support group
		Music	Television

some that did not work for you. The important thing is to find what is comfortable for you and to do it on a daily basis.

With chronic illness, your body is constantly stressed. In addition, emotional and social stresses are multiplied when living with illness on a daily basis. You, more than the average person, need a *daily* means of recovery from the stress spiral—emotional maintenance that impacts on your physical maintenance.

19

New Year's Resolutions

It is often said that New Year's resolutions are made only to be broken. Did you ever make any resolutions? Did you write them down? Did you calculate their cost in time or effort, or plan how you might go about implementing them? Or did they just quickly cross your mind? Perhaps you have already broken them?

One resolution beneficial for the chronically ill is to learn all you can about stress, as it relates to you, individually, and to do all you can to deal with it better. Stress, very simply, is any event produced by a stressor that causes the individual to have to adapt in some way.

Stress can be caused by pleasant as well as unpleasant events, although stress caused by unpleasant events seems to stay around longer and to cause more problems. Stress is an unavoidable, integral, necessary part of life. If managed properly, it can be a friend; if ignored, a fatal enemy.

Stress is experienced both emotionally and physically. With stress, actual changes occur in the chemical balance of the body. The two responses cannot be separated. A change of temperature, a loud noise, success or failure, pain or pleasure, overstimulation or boredom, expectations, belief systems, diet, lifestyle—almost anything in life can produce stress.

Too much stress over a period of time can translate into illness as the body continuously tries to adapt, eventually exhausting its limited resources of adaptation energy. Stress of a biological or emotional nature is also known to exacerbate and prolong disease activity in many chronic illnesses that may have initially been triggered by stress.

Stress can become such a way of life that it is soon indistinguishable and its effects no longer recognized. You may even become addicted to stress.

You may be unaware of stress points in your life and not even know what it is like to really relax.

Stress is an individual matter. What causes stress for one person might not affect the next person. Likewise, stress management is an individual matter that must be tailored to each person's particular needs. One formula won't work for all people. Stress management can be approached in many ways, either through prevention or by dealing with the stress by-products after the stress has occurred.

Social and personality engineering are techniques that can be used to minimize or reduce the frequency of the stress response by reducing the number of things that might trigger it. *Social engineering* takes a close look at what in your lifestyle produces unnecessary stress, such as balance of work and recreation, scheduling, diet, life events entailing environmental and social interaction, and so on. Sources of stress from your environment and social interaction can be modified or avoided.

Your lifestyle is the "roadmap" for living that you adopt early in life through trial–and–error because it works for you. Your lifestyle dictates your self-esteem, your goals in life, and how you approach the three major tasks of life: social relationships, intimate relationships, and career. As you go through life, it can be helpful to assess how well your lifestyle is working for you without causing unnecessary stress.

Personality engineering deals with the way you look at things, the meanings that you attach to events, and your expectations of others and life in general. An event may be neutral or stress-producing, depending on how the information at hand is perceived, evaluated, and given meaning by you.

Your lifestyle is determined by the beliefs you formed early in life as you found out what worked for you and made you happy, and what didn't. You may have come to believe that, to be happy, you needed to control everything, be a perfectionist, please everyone, be a martyr or victim whom everyone else had to take care of.

Feelings, emotions, and defenses play a part here. Becoming aware of and changing or modifying your perceptions, expectations, or beliefs can turn a potentially stressful event with physical arousal into a neutral event producing little or no stress.

Techniques to minimize the intensity of the stress response and to reduce emotional reactivity would include things like meditation, biofeedback, and relaxation techniques. This could be compared to replacing a hair trigger on a gun with one more difficult to squeeze off a shot.

Arousal is reduced, a quiet sense of control is promoted, self-awareness surfaces, and eventually attitudes, perceptions, and behavior are also influenced. The person still experiences stress arousal, but less readily, and recovers from it more quickly.

Techniques to utilize or burn off your stress by-products, wastes, and toxins after stress has occurred, and to promote body consciousness or awareness of your body, are egovoid or noncompetitive physical exercise and body awareness activities. Stress of any kind signals your body to prepare for physical action, even when there may be no appropriate physical response.

Psychosocial stressors that you encounter daily in being part of a family, an employee or employer, or just a human being, usually involve no physical activity. Stress by-products, wastes, and toxins build up in your system and can only be burned off by physical activity or exercise. It might take days for the wastes and toxins caused by a brief argument to be absorbed and flushed from your body without some physical action.

If exercise is noncompetitive or ego involvement is absent, interaction can take place between your body and mind. Adequate exercise of this nature can produce a sense of deep relaxation. It will also burn off stress toxins and wastes, as well as "loop back" to reduce your emotional reactivity and minimize the intensity of your stress response.

SUMMARY

You can take some of these measures and turn them into "New Year's resolutions." They won't solve every problem for you, but any gain is worth the effort. The stress of illness and pain is enough to endure by itself. Why allow more illness to be generated by stresses that you can actively reduce, through your own self-awareness and stress management?

20

Social or Lifestyle Engineering

"I'm sorry, but I can't give you any more medication. Although what you are experiencing is frustrating and painful, at this point it isn't life-threatening and doesn't warrant the side effects that more or different medication would include. To some degree, you'll just have to learn to live with it, change your lifestyle, and see if that helps."

These are words wisely and thoughtfully uttered by a doctor—hard for you to accept and even harder to implement, but not impossible.

One way this advice can be implemented is through social or lifestyle engineering. Your life and environment are full of things that cause stress. Stress can be a by-product of societal, interpersonal, occupational, family, academic, physical (caused by purely biological mechanisms such as exercise, heat, cold, diet, noise, smoke), and other stresses. Social or lifestyle engineering implies a willful, calculated change of lifestyle and / or general environment, in an effort to alter exposure to sources of stress, thus taking command of your life.

The primary goal is *not* to bring about changes in what causes you stress, but instead, to modify your position in relationship to the stressors. For example, if you find it particularly stressful to relate to or work with a particular person, you have three options: to change the amount of time you spend with him, to seek some distance from him, or to remove yourself completely from all involvement with him.

"Lifestyle engineering may be as simple as getting out of bed earlier or driving to work by a different route, or as complex as choosing a profession, a mate, or life goal" (Girdano and Everly, 1979, p. 21). You may have the misconception that you *have* to live a stress-filled life. In reality, you may actively seek out a stressful lifestyle because it offers more money or prestige than one with less stress.

Maybe you haven't considered any substitute for your present way of life. You may fear an alternative more than you fear the consequences inherent in your present lifestyle. *You do have a choice*, but it may take some real soul-searching and setting out of different priorities.

Two basic reasons may deter you from considering social engineering strategies. First, consciously reducing life's stressors may be misinterpreted as running away from that stress which carries a negative connotation in our "stand and fight, John Wayne society." A second reason might be found in the attitude of "it can't happen to me," and a total lack of awareness of your unhealthy stress reactions.

Avoiding stress can be carried to an unhealthy extreme, like wrapping one's self in cotton batting and withdrawing from life. The ideal is for you to seek a balance somewhere in between total disregard for the effects of stress and total escape from stress.

Social engineering strategies are designed to reduce the stress in your life by taking the path of least resistance. To alleviate stress, you have to be able to pinpoint its source and why it is stressful for you.

Stress may be generated when you have to constantly use adaptation energy because of the swings and changes in your life. Frustration breeds stress. Overload as well as deprivation or boredom both result in stress. Stress arises from your biological and ecological existence. However, you can approach each of these areas of life with specific strategies.

Changes or novelty produce *adaptive stress*. Balance and rhythm are essential for a healthy body. Adaptive stress can be avoided or modified by synchronizing biological rhythms with your behavior and establishing set routines and patterns of behavior. Biological rhythms may wax and wane more erratically with the chronically ill. This may make it necessary for you to learn to listen to the familiar messages your body sends, new illness-related messages, and respond to them with appropriate behavior and schedule changes. A new "normal" is then established.

The goal is to have your social clock in rhythm with your biological clock. Setting routines and behavior patterns provide a framework by which to balance your life and reduce stress. As routines become automatic, you use less psychic and physical energy. You should reserve specific time periods for certain tasks on a daily or weekly basis. Set aside one day of the week as "mental health day," making it as simple and relaxing as possible.

Vacations in themselves may produce stress for you. They entail a change of location and scenery, requiring adaptive energy. Don't rely on a vacation to reduce your stress. When your life is already full of turmoil and change, avoid or minimize other changes, if possible. Look at the accumulative effect of the many individual stressors in your life, and see which ones can be eliminated or modified.

Frustration, which explains much of the stress in this country, arises when a desired goal or behavior is inhibited. To understand the source of frustration for you, you must understand why the goal or behavior is desirable or what its rewards are. This gets into fulfilling your basic lifestyle patterns as one who needs to control, be a perfectionist, please, be a martyr or victim.

With this information in mind, alternative behaviors or goals may be considered. The goal or behavior has to be spelled out in concrete terms. For example, you can't just want to be happy, but must decide what concrete things, people, or events make you happy or meet your needs as a part of your overall lifestyle or way of approaching life. Several alternatives may have to be explored.

Overload occurs when there are excessive demands on you and stimulation that triggers your stress response. Time pressure, excessive responsibility or accountability, lack of support, and excessive expectations all play a role in overload. Effective time management, where priorities are set and tasks are efficiently scheduled, can help you to relieve time pressure.

Learning to say "no" and delegating responsibility may be difficult because you may be giving up prestige and power. However, in the long run, this may help you to reduce overload. Enlisting the help of others, accepting fallibility of yourself and others, knowing your optimal stress, and avoiding your individual sources of overload may help reduce or even prevent overload.

Deprivation or boredom produces stress because of lack of stimulation. The chronically ill, in particular, should recognize that there will be times when activities may have to be cut back and boredom will result. By planning ahead and having relaxing activities to engage in during these times, you may avoid boredom.

Activities that are not mentally complex and involve no ego involvement produce relaxation. Relaxation techniques may be needed if you are one of the "racehorses" of life born to run through life. Self-examination and the help of counseling may be required before you can successfully manage tension.

Biological and ecological stresses are by-products of your own bodily rhythms, nutrition, and noise in your environment. By keeping your activities in tune with the rhythms of your body, energy expenditures are maximized. Reducing the intake of sodium, caffeine, junk foods, processed flours, and refined sugars will help provide a less stress-prone diet.

Noise can be a source of physical and psychological stress. Research shows that noise can produce cardiovascular changes, tissue damage in the hearing mechanism, an increase in stress hormones, reduced concentration, and lowered frustration thresholds. With planning, you can alter each of these areas to produce a healthier existence.

SUMMARY

Learning to take charge of yourself may produce a whole new thinking process that can prove difficult. Too often, the "musts" "shoulds," "oughts" and "have tos" of society dictate your reality. Instead, you need to really listen to, know, and accept yourself. With chronic illness becoming a part of your life, you may need to get acquainted with a strange body that responds in a totally unpredictable fashion from what you are accustomed to. You may have to get to know the "new you."

Real freedom comes from a knowledge of yourself—your own physical needs, the way you effect others, how the behavior of other people influences you. Only by learning the boundaries of your freedom do you gain control of your destiny. ". . . Ye shall know the truth, and the truth shall set you free" (John 8:32, KJV).

21

Personality Engineering

Personality engineering is the intentional alteration of stressful aspects of your personality. Your personality is a composite of your values, attitudes, and behavior patterns. Hans Selye believes that, "By adopting the right attitude toward life, one can turn harmful distress into positive stress" (Girdano & Everly, 1979, p. 144).

Your vision of the world and life influences your perceptions, attitudes, meanings, and interpretations you give to situations in life and how you respond to life. It also controls the quality of your participation in life. The nature of your personality and chosen lifestyle is shaped by that vision and results in a habitual outlook on and response to life.

Most of the stress you experience is a result of flaws in the vision that shapes your personality. Your expectations in life are also by-products of your vision of life. If your vision is in line with the realities of your life situation, your expectations will also be more realistic.

In turn, with realistic expectations there will be reduced stress and greater participation in the wholeness of a full and happy human life. To the extent that you are blind or have distorted reality, your life and happiness are diminished.

Lifestyle values provide a system of evaluation, beliefs, and attitudes about the realtive worth of a person, place, or thing. Values are learned at an early age and are pretty rigid and inflexible. The value you attribute to yourself is called self-esteem.

Underrating yourself and constantly focusing on the negative aspects of your life are two common sources of poor self-esteem. Distortions in how you see other people, life, the world, and God are usually traceable to some distortion in the way you see yourself (Powell, 1976, p. 107).

Albert Ellis, a pioneer in rational emotive therapy (RET), feels that all emotions and psychological problems can inevitably be traced back to irrational or illogical thinking and ideas. He contends that "people are not emotionally or psychologically disturbed by events or things but by the views they take of those events or things" (Powell, p. 17). Ellis made a list of eleven erroneous ideas or beliefs that are most commonly found in emotionally and psychologically disturbed people. Each idea or belief represents the predominant lifestyle you've chosen. Anxiety seems to develop predominantly from the first seven ideas, and hostility from the final four:

1. I must be loved and appreciated by everyone in my community, especially those who are most important to me (need to please).
2. I must be perfectly competent, adequate, and successful before I can see myself as worthwhile (perfectionist).
3. I have no control over my happiness—it is completely controlled by external circumstances (victim-discouraged).
4. My past experiences and events of my life have determined my present life and behavior—the influence of the past cannot be changed (victim-discouraged).
5. There is one right and perfect solution to each of my problems. If it is not found, it will be devastating for me (perfectionist).
6. Dangerous or fearful things are causes for great concern and I must be prepared for the worst by constantly dwelling and agonizing over them (martyr / victim).
7. I should be dependent on others and have people stronger than myself on whom I can rely (victim).
8. If life does not work out the way I had planned, it will really be terrible. When things go badly for me, it is a catastrophe (martyr).
9. It is easier to avoid certain difficulties and responsibilities than to face them (controller).
10. Some people are bad, wicked, and villainous and should be blamed and punished (martyr).
11. I should be very upset over the problems and disturbances of other people (martyr).

Ellis categorizes these elven major false beliefs or ideas into three groups, the "three whines," in which something is "awfulized":

1. Poor me!—"awfulizes" one's self
2. Poor, dumb other people!—"awfulizes" what others are doing to me
3. Poor, dumb life and universe!—"awfulizes" what the world is doing to my life situation.

The first thing required for discovering your vision and its distortions is a willingness to face facts, whatever they may be. It is not easy to say you were wrong. On a greater scale, you must be able to admit to a lesser or greater credibility gap between who you really are and who you pretend you are or have illusions of being.

You may be afraid to live in the light of who you really are and to let the illusionary person die. Courage and humility are needed. Silence and solitude are also necessary to come into contact with your vision, but you must act on your insights to make them permanent fixtures in your life.

Victor Frankl, the Jewish psychiatrist referred to earlier, suggests that another essential ingredient in discovering your vision is letting life question you. For instance, the ugly, needy person asks what limits you put on your love; an enjoyable experience asks how capable you are of enjoying life; suffering asks if you believe you can grow and go through hard times. In seeing how you respond to these questions, you are given a candid picture of your vision.

Your perceptions are what make you fragmented or whole, and produce stress or peace. Health is basically an inner attitude, a life-giving vision. Even with a chronic illness you can still be whole, if your vision of life produces healthy attitudes and beliefs. There can be no real change or growth until or unless your basic perception of reality and your vision are changed.

SUMMARY

Your life is in your own hands. Because of this, you can change. Growth is a gradual procedure, sometimes resulting in pain, since you have to let the old die in order for the new to bud into life. You may experience the pain of changed relationships, lifestyle, and self-image in the birthing process, as you individuate and become your own person. Only the truth can set you free, as you become more aware of the validity of your vision's contents, discover its distortions, and replace faulty perceptions with those that are true!

22

Personality Engineering Techniques

Your personality determines your lifestyle and thereby how you handle life events, producing or reducing stress. Some psychologists feel that the basis for personality is formed by the age of five and can't be changed. Other psychologists feel that insight into your personality can lead to an awareness that helps you to "redecide" your lifestyle and approaches to life.

The major personality-related causes of stress are: self perception, "Type A" behavior, and anxious reactivity. You can approach each of these personality-related causes of stress with specific strategies. You need to be honest with yourself in order to see and admit these aspects of your personality. This will enable you to go beyond them.

SELF CONCEPT

The way you feel about yourself, your self-concept or self-esteem, is perhaps one of the greatest factors influencing your behavior, personal stress, and stress management. Research shows that the devalued, helpless, and hopeless self-concept (a totally passive and dependent role within its environment) produces increased stress that can lead to illness.

Viewing and accepting yourself as a blend of your total being, with strengths and weaknesses, and embracing all aspects of yourself as just part of your being (without labeling them as good or bad), is one of the most "wholing/healing" experiences to be had in life. This is not a one-time experience, but an ongoing renewal of self-accepting and loving. It is a lifelong process that adds greater enrichment as time goes by.

A positive self-concept makes a difference in whether a person survives or succumbs to the same illness. A poor self-concept can result from underrating yourself and focusing on the negative aspects of your life. Positive verbalization, accepting compliments, and assertiveness training are three strategies found to be successful in increasing your self-esteem.

Realistic, positive verbalization reinforces your self-concept by pointing out positive aspects about yourself. This can be done by writing such positive messages on a calendar or on notecards in a conspicuous place where they can be seen and reviewed. Simply accepting a compliment without detracting statements of humility, but instead adding statements of agreement, will improve self-esteem.

Assertiveness lays the groundwork for you to really appreciate yourself and to think more positively about yourself (Girdano & Everly, 1979, p. 144). Assertiveness lies somewhere between being passive and aggressive. Assertiveness can be practiced in daily contacts, such as greeting others, giving compliments, using "I" statements to own how you feel, asking "why?", spontaneously expressing feelings, disagreeing with someone when you feel he is wrong, and maintaining eye contact.

An assertive response contains three parts. In the empathy statement, you acknowledge the desires or opinions of the other people. The content statement conveys your own position and its rationale. The action part expresses what you really want done or not done. The sentence map would go something like, "I understand that you . . .", "but I . . .", "therefore, I am going to . . .".

"TYPE A" PERSONALITY

This type of personality includes characteristics such as an intense sense of time urgency; aggression that, at times, evolves into hostility; an intense achievement motive; and polyphasic behavior (where multiple tasks are undertaken at one time).

"Type A" personality is "not a stress response or a stressful situation, but a style of behavior that constantly elicits the stress response which, to a large extent, leads to cardiovascular arousal" (Girdano & Everly, p. 110). Heart problems are seen more often in people with "Type A" personality, secondary to physical changes that occur with increased and prolonged stress.

Time management is a strategy aimed at reducing the sense of time urgency. Allocating blocks of time for and setting up priorities as to the order in which tasks should be tackled are possible means of time management. Making lists of tasks to be done and assigning them to specific days can help. Rewarding yourself when tasks are finished also helps reduce stress.

An overactive ego or heightened ego involvement in what you are doing gives rise to hostility in the "Type A" person. It is helpful to realize that the work is separate from you. It is acceptable not to have all the answers, and it is only human to make mistakes. Everything related to your work is not necessarily directly related to you.

Polyphasic behavior creates stress because the nervous system is stimulated by several sources at once. Instead of being an efficient use of time, it creates anxiety, causes confusion, and often leads to mistakes. Developing the ability to concentrate on one thing while focusing purely on the mechanics of a task, and not constantly analyzing performance, helps alleviate this behavior.

ANXIOUS REACTIVE PERSONALITY

An individual with this type of personality seems to experience stress over an event that lingers long after the event. The stress might even increase. If you are prone to this reaction, you can be mentally and physically incapacitated by even the slightest stress. You can also develop psychosomatic disorders as a result.

Bodily responses to thoughts due to stress serve as a feedback loop and generate greater anxiety. Your thoughts can provide one of the most volatile feedback loops by "catastrophizing" or "reliving" an event over and over after it has happened.

In catastrophizing, you see the event as being far worse than it is. Reliving means you relive any and all crises over and over again in your mind, for days and weeks afterwards, suffering distress every time. If you combine catastrophizing and reliving, you really have an ever-escalating stress spiral.

Thought-stopping is a process where you deliberately try to break the vicious cycle of obsessional thoughts. One method is shouting either to yourself or out loud, "Stop!", as soon as you become aware that you are reliving or catastrophizing.

Another method is to immediately switch your focus to a pleasant scene. The same scene should be used each time, focusing on it for thirty to sixty seconds. You continue to break the cycle until it remains broken, no matter how many times a method has to be used. This can be a powerful tool, but it does take practice.

SUMMARY

Redecision is a beginning. You find a new ability to command your life—to experience your new, free self with excitement, enthusiasm, and energy. Changing personality traits takes a long time, but it can be both successful and rewarding. Replacing stressful behaviors with consistent patterns of constructive behaviors that are less stressful will be rewarding and lead to a healthier, happier life, despite the presence of chronic illness.

You can only discover new possibilities by breaking down old barriers. It's your choice: Only you can decide to "redecide!!!"

23

Replacing the Hair Trigger

"I don't know why, but I seem to fly off the handle at the slightest thing. I feel so wound up—I could just explode!" Have you ever felt like that? If so, you are a normal person under a lot of stress. You can become like a hair trigger on a gun, going off at the slightest pressure when stress mounts up.

Everyone experiences a stress spiral, where each successive stressor sends you a little higher on the stress scale. You become less able to recover from stress arousal and find it hard to relax. Living with a chronic illness on a daily basis adds its own unique stresses while, at the same time, lowering your abilities to cope with any stress. It takes less to cause you stress. A multifaceted dilemma emerges.

The hair trigger on a gun needs to have its spring loosened to help reduce its sensitivity. The intensity of the stress response can be reduced and the emotional reactivity cooled down through relaxation techniques. Meditation, biofeedback, deep muscle relaxation, and breathing exercises are a few techniques that can be used to increase your stress threshold and improve your stress recovery.

MEDITATION

The use of meditation goes back some 7,000 years in history. Most religions advocate some form of meditation. The key element of all meditation techniques seems to be a breaking of thoughts, since thoughts produce emotional and physiological arousal. Meditation is similar to staring into space, with your mind thrown out of gear. However, it is attained intentionally and maintained for a period of time.

Attention is focused on a stimulus that has little arousal for you, allowing feverish thinking to slow down, and producing a calmer, more centered consciousness. The focus is different from person to person and from time to time in the same individual, due to changes in what produces arousal. Your spirit and body are united in a sense of wholeness and presentness, as the "noise" of life is quieted.

The body's physiological responses have been measured during meditation. The body's basic metabolic rate is reduced 16% to 17%, carbon dioxide elimination increases, the respiratory rate decreases, oxygen is used more efficiently, and blood lactate levels that produce anxiety are decreased. Heart rate and blood pressure both drop. Galvanic skin response decreases, reflecting the decreased metabolic rate. These changed responses carry over to other times of the day, blunting and reducing your response to arousal.

There are equally impressive psychological responses. Meditators respond to stress just like anyone else, but recover from stress arousal better and don't get caught in the stress spiral. There seems to be a greater sense of aliveness and responsiveness, while paying less for being so alive. In Eastern thought, meditation broadens perception, allowing the person to "get outside" the ego, decreasing the need to be important. This need is often a big source of stress.

Through meditation, a greater sense of self-love, celebration of life, patience, perspective, and lessened agitation (resulting in peace) may be generated. Indians think of the mind as a drunken monkey, a producer of useless thoughts and internal noise that excludes awareness. The purpose of meditation is to get you past the ego, quiet the chatter of life, and open you up to a new awareness of the universe.

Dr. Herbert Benson, a Harvard cardiologist, has developed in his study on meditation a relaxation response that he feels produces the same effects as meditation. The response involves concentration on breathing patterns while saying the word "one" to yourself upon exhalation. He contends that the full effect of the relaxation response won't be felt until it is used for a month, one to two times a day for ten to twenty minutes. (See Appendix A (page 155).

DEEP MUSCLE RELAXATION

Every time you think of carrying out a motion, the muscles that would actually be involved tense up in an abortive effort, leaving muscle tension behind. The vocal chords move when you are thinking. When stressed, tension shows up in your muscles and you may find yourself exerting needless muscle tension to accomplish a task. Excess muscle tension can be an expression of stress, as well as a cause of stress for you. "Much of the harmful, stress-producing muscle tension is extremely subtle and almost impossible to detect" (Girdano & Everly, 1979, p. 201).

As far back as hundreds of years ago, disease has been connected with inordinate muscle tension. It is only since the end of the last century that systematic relaxation programs have been formulated. Anxiety and tension from everyday stress, coupled with the stresses of chronic illness, can make you an anxious individual whose body adapts by maintaining a chronic state of muscle tension.

Muscular tension by itself can contribute to and worsen physical condition, not to mention the draining effect it has on energy levels. Since the muscular system is involved in every body process and every emotional expression, it follows that muscular relaxation beneficially affects the health of the mind and body.

You may not even be aware of the difference between being tense and being relaxed. There are many different types of muscular relaxation techniques, all of which have the basic goal of teaching you how to relax muscles at will. To do this, you first have to be taught to feel the difference between being tense and relaxed. Some people may be wound so tight that they need to do deep muscular relaxation before they can attempt any meditation techniques. See Appendix B (page 163).

BREATHING EXERCISES

When stressed, the natural rhythm of breathing is interrupted. Hyperventilation or hypoventilation may result. With hyperventilation, breathing is rapid and shallow, resulting in increased oxygen intake and decreased carbon dioxide. Dizziness, weakness, the numbness of an extremity, nervousness, and many other frightening physical responses may result. With hypoventilation, breathing is too slow, resulting in decreased oxygen intake and increased carbon dioxide. Increased oxygen makes the body too alkaline; increased carbon dioxide makes it too acid. At its best, the body is somewhere in between the two and in balance.

The philosophy of yoga contends that the mind is master of the senses, while the breath is master of the mind. The use of breathing exercises results in strengthening and conditioning your pulmonary system, enhancing your cardiovascular system function, promotion of oxygenation, and a calming of your nerves, resulting in restfulness.

The reticular activating system (RAS) is the part of your brain that filters any stimuli reaching the brain. It decides if a stimulus should go any further or be blocked—sort of a "security system" for the brain. "The breathing centers in the brain have a close relationship with the reticular activating system; therefore, constant, steady, restful breathing promotes relaxation" (Girdano & Everly, p. 204).

In addition to promoting neuromuscular relaxation, breathing exercises also play a vital role in the prevention of respiratory ailments. Breathing exercises can help vitalize your lungs' functioning and regulate your breathing patterns, building up respiratory reserves as well as increasing the ability to get oxygen to the blood and body. Prescribed breathing techniques will restore your body to its natural balanced pH condition and relieve nervousness and anxiety. See Appendix C (page 167).

SUMMARY

Your stress spiral can be broken, providing recovery and relaxation by using any or all of these techniques. Each technique may not be appropriate for every person, but you won't know this until you try. The technique must be a comfortable one for you.

The "kettle of life" may begin to boil a little less feverishly as your stress is defused. You may find that you don't have to scrape yourself off the ceiling quite as often. It takes intentional effort and planning for you to incorporate a change into your lifestyle.

24

Me . . . Exercise?!

"What do you mean, exercise?! Here I have a chronic illness! I get tired just walking to the mailbox! You can't know what this fatigue is really like! I'd rather save my energy for other things!" Have you ever given these responses when encouraged to exercise? Let's take a look at some of the pros and cons of activity and inactivity.

Fatigue can actually breed fatigue. Fatigue *from* your chronic illness can actually cause fatigue *of* chronic illness. "Inactivity progressively inhibits the functioning of the autonomic nervous system. The blood circulates more slowly, the poisons in the blood are not oxidized and the system becomes more sluggish" (Jackson, 1979, p. 74).

Technological advances have brought about an increase in mental activity and a decrease in physical activity that can lead to degenerative disease. At the same time, it has become increasingly difficult to deal with the mental overload brought on by technological advances. It is impossible for you to remain in optimum health by performing only sedentary tasks. Physical activity is a natural way of staying as healthy as possible, as well as a way of reuniting your mind/body connection.

BODILY CHANGES
WITH STRESS

When you are stressed, your body is automatically mobilized to prepare for physical activity—to either stand your ground and fight, or turn and run in flight. Your body's responses to stress include: an increase in the supply of blood sugar and fat to the muscles and brain; dilated pupils; increased heart rate; faster and deeper breathing; increased blood pressure; tense and contracted muscles, resulting in an accumulation of pyruvic and lactate acid; blanched skin; and excretion of norepinephrine into the system.

"Norepinephrine causes anxiety until appropriate action is initiated to burn it off" (Girdano & Everly, 1979, p. 222). Research indicates that athletes actually experience *less* harmful stress than spectators because they burn off the stress by-products with activity. Stress causes your body to strip its gears to prepare for action. "If you sit passively when you were meant to move, these stress chemicals will eat at your vital organs and systems" (Matheny, 1981, p. 6).

BENEFITS OF ACTIVITY

Usually, fitness and health go together, but it is possible to have a serious health problem and be physically fit in terms of muscle strength, cardiovascular endurance, and flexibility. "Being fit has the added advantage of reducing the stressfulness of certain physical demands placed on you, of reducing fatigue and the resulting emotional distress" (Matheny, p. 1).

Recent studies show a correlation between regular exercise and improvement in depression, anxiety, hostility, social interaction, and outlook for the future. It seems that exercise can play an important role in improving your self-image. A sense of mastery over the body is also gained, decreasing fear (Cardenas & Kutner, 1982, p. 339).

AEROBIC EXERCISE

Aerobic means "within your breath." Aerobic exercise is exercise performed at the level where no more oxygen is used than is available. Roughly the same amount of oxygen being taken in by the body is being burned up. When exercising anaerobically, an oxygen debt is incurred, producing fatigue and sore muscles. Aerobic exercise is gauged by your pulse rate based on age and other factors.

Aerobic exercise increases the blood supply to the heart. As your heart becomes stronger with use, the heart muscle increases slightly, and capillary growth also increases. Your heart gets more rest, since it is stronger and requires less beats. The production of hemoglobin, which carries oxygen in the blood, is increased, thus increasing the capacity of your respiratory system to exchange oxygen and carbon dioxide, causing a highly energizing effect.

PHYSICAL ACTIVITY AND STRESS

Physical activity provides treatment for and plays a preventive role in managing stress. Treatment is provided by burning off stress products that might otherwise be harmful and contribute to degenerative disease. The preventive role lies in the lessening of arousal after exercise, producing an altered centered mental state. In addition to strengthening your heart, "the working muscles, the hormonal system, metabolic reactions, the responsiveness of the central nervous system, and all the systems are improved in like manner with physical activity, strengthening your ability to cope" (Girdano & Everly, 1979, p. 224).

There is a certain imperturbability, a reduced resting reactivity to the environment, experienced by a regular exerciser. Reaction to stimuli may be more appropriate. The steps may be lighter, the attitude more positive, and it may take more to become upset.

Exercise causes the anterior lobe of the pituitary gland to secrete the body's own natural morphine that is six hundred times more efficient than synthetic morphine. A good time to do your deep breathing and muscle relaxation exercises and then your relaxation technique is immediately following exercise.

CAUTIONS

What may suit you in the way of activity may not be right for another person. Activity must be individually tailored to the chronically ill. You may be able to do different things at different times and not be able to do them at other times. Absolute bed rest may be required in times of increased disease activity. Aerobic exercise may be possible at another time. It may be best to aim for something in between absolute bedrest and aerobic exercise.

The Zen aphorism, "Gentle is the way," should be remembered. It may take weeks, even months, to build up. The reduction of your stress spiral may also be noticed slowly. Be kind to yourself, and don't expect too much, too soon. This will only add stress.

Remember that activity is, in itself, a stressor. What you are trying to do is to kindle a fire that will increase circulation and burn off its own stress by-products as it burns off others. Exercise should be noncompetitive, even with yourself.

Don't compare what you can and can't do now with what you used to be able to do or what someone else can do. A competitive mind is stressful. Stress levels may be elevated when progress doesn't come as quickly or easily as you might have expected or hoped. Try to refrain from self-evaluation.

Some activity on a regular basis is better than none. It may be wiggling your toes in bed several times a day, passive or active range of motion exercises of the joints, riding a stationary bike, isometric exercises, deep breathing exercises, swimming, walking, exercising in the water, or whatever suits you best at the time.

Joint inflammation may be reduced and further inflammation prevented with non-weight-bearing activity. This creates smoothness or agility. It may take trial–and–error to find what you can and cannot do. With extra activity, you will need extra rest time and increased nutrition to sustain the body.

SUMMARY

There is risk involved in anything you do in life. There is risk in trying to exercise, but there is also risk in remaining inactive. NASA has discovered that even in perfectly healthy people, bed rest can cause dramatic deconditioning. If you go to bed for long periods of time, you actually participate in the aging process. Within eighteen hours of going to bed, the heart gets smaller and blood volume is reduced. After three days, your postural and ambulatory muscles lose muscle tone, get flabby, and start to waste away. Dehydration and calcium loss from the bones also occurs. (NASA, 1983, p. 62).

After prolonged bed rest, you'll feel faint upon getting up, due to a drop in blood pressure. With each day in bed, the condition worsens. After about three days it's pretty firmly entrenched. (NASA, p. 62). The caution seems to be, don't stay totally inactive when feeling bad. You'll shorten your convalescence by trying to get up as soon as possible. Deconditioning is a reversible condition.

You have to weigh the advantages and disadvantages. Above all, you must learn to listen to your body and the messages it sends you. Ask your doctor about some form of exercise and what limits you should observe. It may take a lot of time and patience. Even at that, things will fluctuate. My doctors can testify to what it has and is still taking to find the best activity for me, but I haven't given up. Neither should you. Good luck!!

For a copy of guidelines to physical fitness, see Appendix D (page 169).

25

Holiday Blues

Holidays may be a time of potent family and personal traditions, increased activity, altered demands, togetherness, scrambled schedules, and heightened stress and emotion. Those people already moving more slowly than the general masses due to chronic illness may find themselves even more outdistanced by the quickened pace of holidays. Carefully arranged schedules, made to conserve energy, are tossed aside with the demands of a holiday.

Through the years, you may have established ways of expressing yourself during holidays by the gifts you give, the foods you cook, the time spent with family and friends. These are traditions etched in time that have become a part of your life.

As chronic illness invades life, many of these things might have to be handled in a different way. Holiday customs change slowly through the years, as the family dynamics accommodate the different ages represented. The alterations due to chronic illness come more swiftly. It may be difficult to give up customs that have become extensions of yourself.

The heightened emotions of the holidays may be seen in the extremes of "highs" and "lows"—happiness and depression. Blessings and losses are both magnified. We are thankful for the blessings of love and remembrance. We also become sad as we are vividly reminded of losses—health, goals, ambitions, functions—maybe even loved ones or changed relationships. It can be a sober time for reflection. You might take some time to think about where your life is and what is really important.

Although hospitals send as many patients as possible home for the holidays, home health care and mental health agencies find this to be a time of increased need. Lonely, homebound patients call out in their need as the holidays magnify their plight.

On the other hand, the chronically ill with planned family gatherings may experience travel, exposure to more people than usual, the need to prepare larger meals, more activities, and increased excitement. Any way you look at it, demands on time, energy, and emotional coping are increased.

Why consider all this? Well, maybe you have experienced the "holiday blues." This might be a good time to sit back and evaluate what contributed to them and decide how holidays can be handled better.

A price has to be paid for what you do, either physically or emotionally. You have to decide if what you do is worth the price you will have to pay. Maybe you can do things differently by setting priorities. Maybe you won't have to pay such a high price. Here are just a few suggestions:

Shopping by catalogue from your home can be a real help. Items can be wrapped and mailed directly from the mail order house to the recipient. There are now catalogues for just about anything you can imagine, including food.

Meals can be made more simple by letting each guest bring a dish. If possible, plan family gatherings at someone else's home. If this isn't possible, don't hesitate to delegate some responsibility to others. Recognize your limits and seek out a quiet place to rest, even if it is somewhat embarrassing.

Don't spend the holidays completely alone. Very important is the sharing of them with someone else. Find someone to spend a little time with, even if just on the phone. Whenever possible, capture the magic of the music of the season. Whole meals can be catered, if necessary. Pre-cooked turkeys and hams can be purchased. Find your own unique way to reach out to others, staying within your limits. Be good to yourself on special days and find ways to celebrate holidays as well as every day of the year.

SUMMARY

You can't always choose what your circumstances will be, but you can choose what to do with those circumstances. The gifts of love, peace, celebration, and joy can be yours, whatever your situation.

Holidays bring reminders of freedom, wholeness, hope, and rehabilitation to you throughout the year. Chronic illness may give you an edge during holidays since, by traveling at a slower pace, you can more fully recognize and appreciate, treasure, enjoy, and celebrate precious relationships and all the blessings that are yours.

26

Music Therapy

Throughout the ages, music has been a balm to the wounded spirit and a salve to the ailing body. King Saul, in the Old Testament, called forth David to play his harp to soothe him. Modern-day medicine now uses music as a therapeutic tool. Music can provide a distraction, reducing anxiety and thereby stimulating the release of endorphins, the body's own painkillers.

The language of music vibrates the chords of the soul as nothing else can. Worship, anguish, joy, defeat, victory—the full gamut of emotions can be expressed in music. Music can cross cultural, language, and age barriers to reflect the many-faceted rhythms of life.

The television show, *Real People*, featured a therapy group centering around people singing both individually and as a group. The basic premise for the therapy was that music provided an emotional release, and also served to bind people together. The people expressed jubilation and joy in experiencing music together. Many had moist eyes as they concluded their session.

Music has always had a significant place in my life. Although I can no longer perform as a soloist or choir member, I still find a great deal of emotional expression and enjoyment in music. It has perhaps played an even greater role in my life since chronic illness announced itself and I've had to rearrange my life to fit this piece of furniture in.

Every moment is filled with some kind of music. The amount of disease activity, to some degree, determines the beat I can tolerate. Songs like *I Made It Through The Rain*, sung by Barry Manilow; *Sweet, Sweet Surrender* and *Today*, sung by John Denver; and the theme from the television show, *The Greatest American Hero*, sung by Joey Scarborough, are my "pick-me-ups." They put to music thoughts and themes that have become important in my life. *Climb Every Mountain, The Impossible Dream, Be Thou My Vision, Amazing Grace*, and *God Who Touchest Each With Beauty* echo the songs of my heart.

SUMMARY

Music can soothe and lift the spirit, lance the soul, create vision, and take us beyond where we are. During one hospitalization, I enjoyed playing my John Denver tape and harmonizing with it—while in bed, in the tub, or the hall! It was my high spot on days when I was feeling pretty low! My radio and tape player are "musts" when I pack for the hospital.

27

Me . . . See A "Shrink"?!

"Me . . . see a 'shrink'?!" This is a common reaction to the suggestion that you see a psychiatrist or get counseling. Whether made by a doctor, a family member, a friend, or a pastor, such a suggestion may be taken as criticism or a put-down. It brings with it the connotation that you're somehow weak and unable to cope with things.

There is a deep-seated feeling within you that says you don't need that kind of help. Going to a psychiatrist carries a taboo. Such an experience is not readily talked about.

Regardless of all this, the psychiatrist is a very important member of the medical team that treats the chronically ill patient. It is difficult to admit the need to see a psychiatrist. When you have kidney involvement, it is easier to see the nephrologist; or the dermatologist, if you have skin problems, and so on.

The emotions not only have great control over how you feel and interpret things, but also have an effect on the level of your disease activity in a chronic illness. When experiencing a chronic illness, you might encounter heightened emotions, such as anger, anxiety, or depression.

The added expense of seeing a psychiatrist or getting counseling may be a heavily-weighed factor in deciding whether or not to pursue the referral. Medical expenses may already be sapping your budget. Sometimes you may improve physically, but emotions may remain a problem. Adjustment to a chronic illness is 10% physical and 90% mental. A trip to a "shrink" may actually save on medical bills in the long run.

Physical complaints can overshadow an emotional response so that it can initially be missed. In anxiety and depression, the emotional stress that results can cause rapid heart beat, poor appetite, fatigue, hyperventilation, urinary frequency, insomnia (Harvey, 1972, p. 1445), skin rashes, muscle tension, shortness of breath, diarrhea, constipation, headache, indigestion, hypertension (Holvey, 1972, p. 1369), and many other problems.

It is sometimes difficult for a physician to determine *where* the physical problem relates to the emotional problem, or vice versa. Psychiatry is the branch of medicine that is concerned with the body's function as a whole (Harvey, p. 1444), physical and emotional. The physical, mental, and spiritual are intimately interwoven, each affecting the others.

When I was having a flare that involved respiratory problems, my physician suggested that I see a psychiatrist. My first reaction was one of hurt and anger. I felt I had been coping pretty well with all the turmoil that chronic illness had dumped into my lap.

His suggestion came across to me as saying, "I don't feel you're handling this very well—maybe you need some help." It made me feel that he didn't think my respiratory complaints were based on real, physical problems, but only a manifestation of my anxiety.

Some time elapsed before the actual referral was made. I went back to some of my nursing textbooks and reviewed the overlapping effects the emotions can have on the physical self. Slowly, I began to realize how difficult it is to weed out the intertwined effects of emotions on your physiological functioning. I could see the strain the many adjustments to chronic illness was putting on me, my marriage, and my family life.

As chronic illness and different medications exert their effects, personality changes can occur. With any chronic illness, you have some personality changes. Your personality as it was before becomes magnified, both the good and the bad. You'll be the same as you were before illness, only more so!

If a psychiatrist had never met you and didn't know you prior to changes due to illness or medication, how could he know what behavior was new and what was old? Along with all these other reasons, I realized this might be a chance to grow in self-understanding. Keeping all these things in mind, I decided to see that "shrink"—maybe it was a good idea, after all.

On my first visit, there was no couch to lie on, as I had anticipated, only comfortable sofas to sit on. The atmosphere was very relaxed. For two one-hour sessions, I had the opportunity to open up and share all of the hurts, adjustments, fears, anxieties, worries, hopes and dreams I was experiencing and their relationships to my illness— in a non-stop stream of communication that helped me to put together thoughts that had been fragmented.

The psychiatrist understood the devastating effect that losing control of life has on the ego, the strain of changes made in lifestyle, the fear of the unknown related to illness, and the disrupting effect a sudden hospitalization has on an individual and family unit. Almost every aspect of my life was and would continue changing in some ways.

Very carefully, he picked out small crystals of thought and held them up for me to examine. Looking at them closely, I could see where, in some instances, I was exerting my energy and getting nowhere. He helped me to get a better grasp on things and to cope somewhat better.

I discovered some things about myself. I realized that I do worry a lot, and admitted it to myself. Before, I had always justified it under the guise of something else. By admitting to myself that I do worry, I was also able to acknowledge that worrying never changes anything; it's a futile, self-defeating activity.

I decided to write down everything I worried about. I even worried about worrying! The uselessness of it all dawned on me and helped me to shed some of the worry-shell that I was carrying around with me.

Other aspects of my life became clearer. I recognized that it is very necessary to keep communication lines open; that I'm not responsible for other people's reactions or responses to me, nor can I change them; that I must be myself; that, in ventilating problems, somehow things fall into better perspective; that the effects that emotions have on symptoms related to illness should not be discounted; that some anxiety and depression is normal but should be self-limiting; and that whether from a psychiatrist or other counselors, counseling can help.

If I get into deep water emotionally in the future, whether from my illness, reaction to drugs, or family or social problems, I feel that my psychiatrist knows me and I know him. I wouldn't be going to a stranger. He could better determine what was going on with me.

I left my "shrink's" office with the understanding that I would return if I experienced depression that I couldn't "bounce back" from, if thoughts of my illness and its effects became a preoccupation, or if family problems became difficult. It was up to me.

SUMMARY

Me, see a "shrink?!" You'd better believe it!! I have and continue to call my friend, the "shrink," when I find myself facing too many problems to handle alone, or maybe one big dilemma I can't seem to shake, get around, or through.

My friend, the "shrink," is an important member of my health care team: I have no qualms in others knowing I see him, and even brag about how well he knows me and how much he helps when I need him.

28

A Journey Inward

My world was neatly arranged—everything in order, schedules to live by, plans for the future. I really had it "all together." Hard work was paying off in success and personal fulfillment as a wife, mother, and career woman.

I fancied myself as the "Enjoli Woman," who was able to bring home the bacon, cook it, nurture my children, and still be sexy by the end of the day. Everything seemed almost "too good."

From out of the blue, chronic illness struck and my whole life was transformed right before my eyes. There was no order, schedules were made only to be broken, and plans for the future were replaced by a mist of vague uncertainty.

Just getting up and dressed could be hard work. Sometimes the whole day would be spent just trying to get up. The "Enjoli Woman" became the "Geritol Woman," with tired blood!!!

Days that were once filled with activity were emptied into inactivity. I just existed. Although the body came to a sudden halt, the mind raced about in a futile manner, thoughts bumping into one another, chased about by fear, uncertainty, anger, guilt, and confusion in a marathon fashion.

My life of order had become chaos and I really wasn't sure who I was anymore, without all those plans and scheduled activities to give structure to my days. My list of priorities no longer seemed so important to me.

As a young girl and teenager, I had been a faithful diary keeper, filling a couple of five-year diaries with events, happenings, feelings, and reminiscences of my growing-up years. Young impressions and stages of growth were captured.

Little did I know that, as a youngster, I was developing a practice that would be a major tool to help me maintain and salvage my sanity, find my way in the dark, make it through the storm stirred up by chronic illness back into the sunshine, and even find a rainbow along the way.

Following my instincts, not really knowing what I was doing, I began journaling my thoughts, emotions, and feelings evoked by turbulent events in my changed life, in the form of a prayer diary. My thought patterns were fragmented, distracted, and, at times, obsessional. Journaling was the only way I could make it through a complete prayer thought and lay my soul, wounds, burdens—my very being—at the feet of the Great Physician, to open my arms to His healing/wholing.

Having completely expressed a thought or emotion, worry or anxiety, fear or concern, I can turn to other things, released and freed. I have embarked on an inner journey to find, accept, and love the essence of my being, warts and all, devoid of the hustle and bustle. This sojourn helps "put my life in perspective, find in life some deeper meaning, and discover the subtle 'intimations of truth' that give direction to life" (Kaiser, 1981, p. 64).

While becoming poor in the world's view of what life should be, I am becoming rich in awareness of my inner self. In doing so, I tap into my own inner well-springs of joy, peace, and celebration. "Poverty is not simply the lack of money. Ultimately, it is a person's lack of feeling for the reality of his own inner being" (Kaiser, p. 67).

Repressed or unacknowledged feelings can be lethal to the soul, love, marriage, health, personal freedom, and being. Whether feelings are unconsciously blocked or repressed out of fear, guilt, pity, or some misguided sense of protection of the self or others, makes no difference. Your "shoulds/oughts/musts/have to's" born in childhood and carried into adult life as excess garbage may explain why feelings are held back, only to be expressed in unhealthy, destructive actions. The results are just as deadly, no matter what the unconscious reason.

When out of touch with your feelings, you cease to live fully and experience yourself. You are out of touch with the truth of the reality of your inner being. Feelings and truths about myself that I divorce continually need to be faced, acknowledged, labeled, dealt with, wedded, and integrated as a part of myself. The feelings and accompanying truths descend upon me in torrents, sometimes nearly sweeping me away, but ultimately cleansing and freeing me to be *me*.

I entered the school of learning "to be" rather than "to do." My "shoulds," "oughts," and "musts" were translated into needs, wants, and likes. I found that the "doing" just naturally flowed out of my totally "being," with no effort or exertion.

I am learning to live to the rhythm of my soul's own music, not according to the tunes of oldies from the "good ol' days." The Lord lifted me out of the miry clay and gave me a new song (Psalms 40).

On this lifetime journey that leads to facing the good and the not-so-good of my being, accepting and loving them both, there are times when it isn't easy and I want to run away from it all. "Wherever there is a reaching down into innermost experience, into the nucleus of personality, most people are overcome by fright, and many run away . . . The risk of inner experience, the adventure of the spirit is, in any case, alien to most human beings" (Powell, 1978, p. 8).

Ira Progoff, a psychologist, stumbled upon the benefits of journaling during an emotional crisis in his life. In the upheaval following separation from his wife and the threat of losing his two children, he began writing in a notebook. "He discovered that he was able to get a fix on his life by writing things down, going over them, feeding them back into the computer of his mind, as it were, engaging in a dialogue with himself and with his wife and children" (Kaiser, p. 76).

"Journaling is a catharsis in the best sense" (Pearson, 1965, p. 14) and provides an outlet for emotional expression to a "paper psychiatrist." There may be a sense of greater freedom of expression, knowing that only you will see your thoughts. A blank piece of paper may be less threatening than a staring human face.

You can set your own pace, revise your wording, and, most of all, look at the words you use. "Very often your reactions are determined by the words you use to describe your situation" (Powell, 1976, p. 151). You can gain some control of your thoughts and emotions rather than letting them control you.

The exercise of a daily emotional diary or journal can help "analyze and synthesize an emotion in a deep personal way and, as such, works counter to repressive and regressive forces in the personality. It is a way of development of insight and cognition" (Pearson, p. 14).

Intimacy with the self is promoted, as well as intimacy with others. "The process of growth in a human being, the process out of which the person emerges, is essentially an inward process" that leads to the meaning, truth, and reality of your own inner being (Kaiser, p. 72). Journaling is actually a form of process meditation.

Do not content yourself with merely thinking about what you might write. Thinking about what you'd possibly write is not the same thing as writing it. Writing evokes depth that thinking does not reach. The process meditation procedures give each person a means of taking whatever meaningful experiences they already have in their lives—whether large and dramatic or small and inconspicuous—and using them as starting points for new and often unpredictable, inner events (Progoff, 1980, pp. 22-23).

Very often, if left to yourself, you do not organize and clearly see the pieces of a problem and its ramifications. The problem remains vague and poorly understood. In talking with someone else, things may fall into place more clearly. Journaling is a conversation with the self. It can serve the very same purpose of clarification.

"Obviously, the more precise and vivid the verbalization in writing of this kind, the greater the likelihood that misconceptions will surface for recognition" (Powell, 1976, p. 152). The greater the truthfulness of the description of your feelings, the greater the chance of insight and change.

Activities, events, problems, and spontaneous emotional reactions to them can be written down. Going over what is written and reexamining it can help "check out and challenge the validity of the belief system or vision between events and the emotional reaction to it" (Powell, 1976, pp. 151-152). In this way, new insights may be gained, emotional patterns may be challenged, and perceptions may broaden as growth occurs and emotional reactions change.

Journaling helps me to untangle the web of my emotions and thoughts that are spun in the midst of confusion and conflict, trapping me. I am freed from the useless ramblings of my feverish mind as I release emotions, see the reflections of my thoughts, and redefine the dimensions of my vision of reality. Order replaces chaos, fears are quieted, uncertainty is cleared up, anger is defused, guilt is recognized, and confusion is replaced by clear thinking. I can leave the struggle of my mind there on that stark piece of white paper and go in peace..

Journaling can act as the catalyst to stir probing thoughts and peel back the layers of deadened feelings, exposing healthy emotions. It can serve as the shovel to remove excess emotional garbage. It can also be the sensor to pick up the impulses of your soul, and the telescope or microscope to visualize the reality of the expanse or the minutia of your emotional truths. You will be led to the bridge of your spiritual and emotional freedom.

You cross over this bridge of freedom as you integrate insights and understandings of your life, giving birth to new beginnings. You may or may not leave anything behind or really change the circumstances of your life. Your inner world is inescapable. It goes with you wherever you go.

All that may change is an awareness of your inner self, allowing you to relate to your world differently, unencumbered by antiquated and inappropriate emotional messages from your past. In this way, you truly learn the celebration-dance of the present moment!

In breaking loose from the prison of confining thoughts and emotions, I can be more open to the spontaneity of the moment, be more creative with what I have left, be more sensitive to those around me and their feelings, be free to love myself and others with greater abandon, and approach life unencumbered by excess emotional garbage. My inward journey ultimately allows me to embrace life in all its fullness, as I continue to struggle with chronic illness and its many challenges on a daily basis.

SUMMARY

Journaling gives me a tool to light the way and to avoid the emotional ruts that lie along the road of life that includes chronic illness. These ruts can make life's trip even rougher than it already is. When troubled or perplexed, I reach for my pen and journal, finding my way through the fog of my mind to some new direction. Vague feelings are defined, wandering thoughts find direction, solutions to problems emerge, and answers to questions become more apparent.

I have become the "Enjotol Woman," who knows her limits but also celebrates her potentials. The two self-images became merged in my journey inward. I find myself a much healthier and happier person to live with. New aspects of my weird, wild, wonderful self continue to emerge from the pages of my journal to greet me. It's an exciting trip!

29

Bibliotherapy

"Me, read a book?! You've got to be joking! I'd rather be out riding my horse, swimming, or playing ball with the guys. Books are boring! Besides, I have too many other things I want to do."

That was pretty much my attitude, growing up on a farm with my own mare I'd raised and trained, a lake, and woods to roam through. In addition, I was too busy trying to keep up with my two older brothers, playing football, baseball, and other sports. A real "Annie Oakley," for sure! Reading seemed like such a waste of time!

This attitude carried over into my adult life. While at Vanderbilt in nursing school, I read *only* the absolutely required material. I was too busy dating the guy I was going to marry.

There was even less time to read after our two sons were born. I worked to put Jim through eight years of school for his master's and doctorate at the seminary, and carried out the many functions of "pastor's wife" and mother. There were always too many other important things to do with my time and energy.

When chronic illness came into my life, the hurry and scurry of life was slowed down, and I found a lot of time on my hands. I didn't have much energy to do anything. I began to realize I had entered a whole new way of living that I knew nothing about. I needed to learn how to exist in this new reality. I began reading everything I could get my hands on.

I noticed things in my emotional being changing in unhealthy ways. I realized that I could learn either healthy adaptive or unhealthy maladaptive illness behavior. My physical illness could translate into an emotional illness if I didn't learn how to live with it in emotionally healthy ways.

Reading turned out to be one of my footholds on stability, as everything in my life seemed to change. Reading not only filled my time; it filled my mind with words of wisdom, comfort, insight, guidance, inspiration, strength, and patience, as I heard the echoes of my own experience captured in the writings of others.

A jewel of thought gleaned from the reflections of others shed light to illuminate and challenge me. Setting my own pace, I began to discern and understand truths about my changed reality and aspects of myself that I had never needed to face before. I got to know a blend of the old and new me.

To Kiss The Joy

This book, written by Robert Raines, was one of the first I read, through the fog of a clouded, confused, and troubled mind. It touched my wounded spirit and continues to bring me joy each time I read it. In it I found what has become my goal for living—"To kiss the joy (life) as it flies is to live in the Spirit, it is to live boldly, immediately, with gracious abandon, daring to risk much, willing to give one's self."

I also found that —"To go with the flow of your life is to live without a map—to be vulnerable to having your mind and plans changed, your heart broken, your dreams fulfilled. It is to trust that God is in the rapids of change as well as in the rocks of continuity. It is being able to stop digging your heels in against the tide of tomorrow."

The joy, life, was symbolized by a fleeting, delicate butterfly. If held too tightly, it would be crushed. Touched lightly, it could bring wonder, peace, blessing, and celebration.

On Borrowed Time

Dr. Samuel Chyatte's book touched me profoundly, as he related his journey with chronic illness. In it I learned—"Denial isn't all bad. I'm sick, but I keep going. I push away all the implications of my illness so I can function today. That's useful denial . . . . Depression and tears seem to be the mechanism that restored the grieved to normalcy. . . .

"All living creatures constantly undergo change. We are influenced by personal experience, by what we read, what we see, our successes, and our failures. Illness, especially chronic illness, is an experience that can alter outlook, our self-image, and our expectations."

His insights into relationships of the chronically ill provided me with a much needed bridge of understanding. He summed it up by saying, "Keep a humorous perspective on your illness that tells your plight and leaves them smiling." With the gut honesty of one who has "been there," he touches on the topics of children, family, doctors, marriage, sex, work, as they become entangled in the web of chronic illness.

Man's Search for Meaning

From Victor Frankl's book, telling of his experience and insights gained from living in a Nazi concentration camp, I reaped these thoughts: "The attempt to develop a sense of humor and see things in a humorous light is some kind of trick learned while mastering the art of living . . . Inner meaning cannot be lost. It is this spiritual freedom—which cannot be taken away—that makes life meaningful and purposeful. . . .

"A man who let himself decline because he could not see any future goal found himself occupied with retrospective thoughts. In robbing the present of its reality lay a certain danger. It becomes easy to overlook the opportunities to make some positives of camp life, opportunities that really did exist. . . .

"It is a peculiarity of man that he can live only by looking to the future . . . sudden loss of hope and courage can have a deadly effect . . . Human life under any circumstances never ceases to have meaning, and that this infinite meaning includes suffering and dying, privation and death."

Getting Well Again

Carl and Stephanie Simonton and James Creighton have written from experience about the effect the psyche has on illness, especially cancer. "We all participate in our own health through our beliefs, our feelings, our attitudes toward life, as well as more direct ways, such as through exercise and diet. The individual who assumes the victim stance participates by assigning meaning to life's events that proves that there is no hope."

"By recognizing your own participation in the onset of your illness, you acknowledge your power to participate in regaining your health and you have also taken the first step toward getting well. . . . It is our central premise that illness is not purely a physical problem, but rather a problem of the whole person, that it includes not only the body, but mind and emotions. Expectancy, either positive or negative, can play a signficant role in determining an outcome."

Bibliotherapy

Unintentionally, I had stumbled onto a type of therapy called bibliotherapy. "The idea of bibliotherapy has been around for centuries. Aristotle said literature aroused emotions that had healing effects; the library of Thebes bore the inscription, 'The Healing Place of the Soul'; the inscription, 'The Medicine Chest of the Soul' is found in the medieval Abbey Library of St. Gall, Switzerland. In its broadest sense, bibliotherapy is defined as the use of literary work in the treatment of physical or emotional problems. Bibliotherapy seeks to change behavior or attitudes" (Fincher, 1980, p. 223).

"Bibliotherapy means guided reading that helps individuals form understandings of the self and environment, learn from others, or find solutions to problems. It consists of three fundamental processes between reader and literature: identification, catharsis, and insight. Identification begins with an affiliation between a reader or a character (or situation) in a story. This identification may expand one's sense of being different from others" (Schrank & Engels, 1981, p. 224).

"Catharsis takes place when readers share and vicariously experience motivations and conflicts presented in literature. Readers often realize their own identification and thus gain insight into motives of their own behavior. Insight occurs when readers see themselves in the behaviors described in the reading material" (Schrank & Engels, p. 224).

"Bibliotherapy is humanizing because through it individuals can see their feelings and needs are similar to others. Symptoms become less frightening when they are discovered to be not uncommon among other people, and there may be emotional release of guilt, anger, depression, or tension" (Fincher, p. 224).

Other objectives of bibliotherapy are:

1. To see that more than one solution to a problem is possible.
2. To see values involved in an experience in human terms.
3. To provide facts needed for the solution of a problem.
4. To provide encouragement to face a situation realistically (Bryan, 1939, p. 774).

This book is bibliotherapy.

SUMMARY

Knowing someone else has experienced similar problems and "made it through the rain" gives you hope, courage, and commitment in order to find your way. Reading books is now an integral part of my survival tactics; it challenges and sustains my living, growing, and stretching of myself. Through reading, I have been invited to grow in ways I never would have otherwise.

Following is a list of books that have brought me special meaning and understanding. You might want to try some of these and look for others that appeal to you. They can help you to live fully with chronic illness.

SUGGESTED BIBLIOTHERAPY READING LIST

Lloyd H. Ahlem, *How to Cope with Conflict, Crisis and Change,* Regal Books.

Les Carter, *Good 'n' Angry,* Baker Book House.

Samuel B. Chyatte, M.D., *On Borrowed Time,* Medical Economics Co.

John Claypool, *In the Steps of a Fellow Struggler*, Word Books.

Gary R. Collins, *The Joy of Caring*, Word Books.

Jan Cox-Gedmark, *Coping with Physical Disability*, The Westminster Press.

Wayne W. Dyer, *Your Errogenous Zones*, Funk & Wagnalls.

Joni Eareckson, *Joni* and *A Step Further*, Zondervan Publishing House.

Albert Ellis, *How to Live With a Neurotic*, Wilshire Book Co.

Victor Frankl, *Man's Search for Meaning*, Beacon Press.

Daniel Girdano & George Everly, *Controlling Stress and Tension . . . A Holistic Approach*, Prentice-Hall.

Sean Hogan, *Coping with Depression in Chronic Illness*, Monograph from the Michigan Lupus Foundation.

Edgar N. Jackson, *The Many Faces of Grief*, Abingdon Press.

Paul E. Johnson, *Healer of the Mind*, Abingdon Press.

Harold S. Kushner, *When Bad Things Happen to Good People*, Avon.

Dennis & Matthew Linn, *Healing Life's Hurts*, Paulist Press.

Myron Madden, *The Power to Bless*, Broadman.

Robert Masters & Jean Houston, *Listening to the Body*, A Delta Book.

Randolph C. Miller, *Live Until You Die*, Pilgrim Press.

Rudolf M. Moos, *Coping with Physical Illness*, Plenum Medical.

Karl Olsen, *Come to the Party*, Word, Inc.

John J. Parrino, Ph.D., *From Panic to Power . . . The Positive Uses of Stress*, John Wiley & Sons.

John Powell, *Fully Human, Fully Alive; He Touch Me; Why Am I Afraid to Tell You Who I Am?; The Secret of Staying in Love; Unconditional Love*, Argus Communications.

Ira Progoff, *The Practice of Process Meditation*, Dialogue House.

W. T. Purkiser, *When You Get to the End of Yourself*, Baker Book House.

Robert Raines, *To Kiss the Joy*, Word Books.

Franklin C. Shontz, *The Psychological Aspects of Physical Illness and Disability*, MacMillan & Co.

O. Carl Simonton, Stephanie Matthews-Simonton, James L. Creighton, *Getting Well Again*, Bantam Books.

Elizabeth Skoglund, *Coping*, Regal Books.

Samuel Standard & Helmuth Mathan, *Should the Patient Know the Truth?*, Springer Publishing Co., Inc.

Earl A. Tooms, *The Self in Pilgrimage*, Harper & Row.

David Viscott, *Risking*, Pennant Books.

Jean A. Werner-Beland, *Grief Responses to Long-Term Illness and Disability*, Reston.

Beatrice A. Wright, *Physical Disability: A Psychological Approach*, Harper & Row.

Appendices

Appendix A

The Relaxation Response is a natural innate protective mechanism which allows us to turn off harmful effects from stress through changes that decrease heart rate, lower metabolism, decrease rate of breathing, and in this way bring the body back into a healthier balance. There are four basic elements necessary to evoke the Relaxation Response:

a. a quiet environment,
b. an object to dwell upon,
c. a passive attitude—"let it happen," and
d. a comfortable position.

In order to trigger the Relaxation Response, follow the steps below:

1. Sit quietly in a comfortable position.
2. Close your eyes.
3. Deeply relax all your muscles, beginning at your feet and progressing up to your face. Keep them relaxed.
4. Breathe through your nose. Become aware of your breathing. As you breathe out, say the word "ONE" silently to yourself. For example, breathe IN . . . OUT, "One": IN . . . OUT, "ONE": etc. Breathe easily and naturally.

5. Continue for 10 to 20 minutes. You may open your eyes to check the time, but do not use an alarm. When you finish, sit quietly for several minutes, at first with your eyes closed and later with your eyes opened. Do not stand up for a few minutes.
6. Do not worry about whether you are successful in achieving a deep level of relaxation. Maintain a passive attitude and permit relaxation to occur at its own pace. When distracting thoughts occur, merely return to repeating "ONE." With practice, the response should come with little effort. Practice the technique once or twice daily, but not within two hours after any meal since the digestive process seems to interfere with the elicitation of the Relaxation Response.

In a comparison study, Dr. Benson found that the physiologic changes elicited by six different techniques (Transcendental Mediation, Zen and Yoga, Autogenic Training, Progressive Relaxation, Hypnosis with suggested deep relaxation, and Sentic Cycles) approximate these changes elicited by the Relaxation Response. The physiologic measurements consisted of oxygen consumption, respiratory rate, heart rate, alpha waves, blood pressure and muscle tension.

Key Religious Equivalents to the Relaxation Response

1. St. Augustine, Martin Luther, Fray Francisco de Osuna, St. Theresa, Father Nicolas, and other early Christian mystics practiced "contemplation" and "recollection" in order to shut off the mind from external thoughts and to produce a passive attitude and mental solitude.
2. Contemplation or meditative exercises are found in early Judaic literature. Merkabolism, the earliest form of mysticism in Judaism, involved repetition of a magic emblem. A 13th Century Rabbi, Abulafia, used the letters of God's name as an object upon which to meditate. He also incorporated yogic breathing and body posture techniques.
3. The Eastern meditative practices have been extremely influential. The best known is Yoga Meditation, the essence of which is concentration on a single point to achieve a passive attitude. Bud-

dhism, Sufism and Taoism, all primarily Eastern religions, contain many elements analagous to Yoga Meditation and thus to the Relaxation Response.

THE MUSCULAR RELAXATION RESPONSE

The relaxation technique you are about to experience is called the "Muscular Relaxation Response." It involves several very simple steps, and takes a total of about 20 minutes to complete. This technique is particularly useful for relaxing and unwinding at the end of a hard, tension-producing day. It has also been helpful with the following problems: sleep difficulties, tension headaches, excessive worrying, and nervousness. You should be in a comfortable and relatively quiet environment: sitting in a chair, on a sofa, or another piece of furniture that allows you to stretch your arms and legs and your entire body to its maximum length. If you think that you can concentrate for 20 minutes without falling asleep, you may lie down on a bed, sofa, or even the floor. It is important for you to complete the relaxation instructions without falling asleep, in order to obtain maximum benefit from the technique. If you wish, you may sleep after the instructions are completed.

Loosen any tight clothing that you may be wearing, like a tie or belt, and if your shoes are uncomfortable, take them off. You are now ready to begin the relaxation technique. You will relax your toes first and then progressively move up to and relax each part of the body until you finish with the face.

1. **Close your eyes and concentrate on your toes:** Curl them down toward the soles of your feet and tense them vigorously— hold that tension for about five seconds. As you count to five, you should tense the toes more and more vigorously. 1—2—3—tighter —4—a little tighter—5. Before letting the tension go, take a deep breath. Let the breath out and release the tension in your toes at the same time. Notice the feeling of relief. Then repeat the word "relax" to yourself. "Relax. Relax. Relax."

2. **With your eyes closed, now concentrate on your calves, the lower part of your legs:** Point your toes up towards your face and tighten your calves vigorously. Hold that tension for about 5 seconds. As you count to 5, you should tense the calves tighter and tighter. 1—2—3—tighter—4—a little tighter—5. Take a deep breath and then let go of the tension in your calves and your breath at the same time. Repeat the word "relax" to yourself. "Relax. Relax. Relax."

3. **Concentrate on your thighs, the upper part of your legs.** Extend your legs out in front of you and point the toes up toward your face once again, this time tightening your thighs vigorously. Hold that tension for about 5 seconds. As you count to 5, you should tense the thighs more and more vigorously. 1—2—3—tighter—4—a little tighter—5. Take a deep breath, and then let go of the tension in your thighs and the deep breath at the same time. Good. Repeat the word "relax" to yourself. "Relax. Relax. Relax."

Notice the difference now between the feelings that you are getting from your legs as compared to the feelings from your upper body. Your legs are more relaxed and heavier, and you may be feeling a tingling sensation from them. Your upper body is tighter. Concentrate on that difference for a moment.

4. **Now, concentrate on your buttocks, or rear end:** Tense them by pushing this part of your body down against the seat of your chair or against the bed or sofa. Push down. 1—2—3—tighter—4—a little tighter—5. Take a deep breath, and let go of the tension in your buttocks and the deep breath at the same time. Good. Repeat the word "relax" to yourself. "Relax. Relax. Relax."

5. **Concentrate on your abdomen or stomach area:** Tense this part of your body by imagining that you are going to protect yourself from a punch or blow coming toward your stomach. O.K., tense your abdomen. 1—2—3—tighter—4—a little tighter—5. Take a deep breath. Hold it for a second and then let go of the tension in your stomach and the breath at the same time. Very good. Repeat the word "relax" to yourself. "Relax. Relax. Relax."

6. **Concentrate on your chest:** Tighten your chest by clasping your hands together—the palm of one hand pressing against the palm of your other hand. Press them together. 1—2—3—harder—4—a little tighter—5. Take a deep breath. Hold that for a second; and, now, let your hands go from each other very slowly. Let your breath out at the same time. Good. Repeat the words "relax" to yourself. "Relax. Relax. Relax."

7. **Concentrate on your shoulders:** Tighten your shoulders by shrugging them, bringing your head down between your shoulders as far as it will go. Shrug your shoulders. 1—2—3—tighter—4—a little tighter—5. Take a deep breath. Hold the breath for a second. Now slowly let go of the tension in your shoulders and let your breath out at the same time. Good. Repeat the word "relax" to yourself. "Relax. Relax. Relax."

8. **Concentrate on your arms:** Extend them out in front of you, tighten your fist, and tense the upper portion of your arms and your forearms together. 1—2—3—tighter—4—a little tighter—5. Take a deep breath. Now slowly let go of the tension in your arms and the breath at the same time. Repeat the word "relax" to yourself. "Relax. Relax. Relax."

9. **Concentrate on your throat:** Tighten your throat by pressing your chin down against the upper part of your chest. Press down vigorously. 1—2—3—harder—4—a little harder—5. Take a deep breath. Let both the tension in your throat and the breath out at the same time. Repeat the word "relax" to yourself. "Relax. Relax. Relax."

10. **Concentrate on the back of your neck and head:** Tense the back of your neck and head by pressing your head down against the back of your shoulders. Press hard. 1—2—3—harder—4—a little harder—5. Take a deep breath. Let the tension and breath out at

the same time. Good. Repeat the word "relax" to yourself. "Relax. Relax. Relax."

11. **Concentrate on your face—your forehead, eyes, nose, cheeks, mouth, and chin:** Tense these areas of your face by making a funny face. Wrinkle your forehead, close your eyes tightly, and grit your teeth at the same time. Tense your face. 1—2—3—tighter—4—a little tighter—5. Take a deep breath. Let the breath and tension go. Now, make another funny face—wrinkle your forehead, open your eyes wide, and open your mouth as big as it will open. Stretch your face. 1—2—3—tighter—4—a little tighter—5. Take a deep breath. Let the breath and tension go. Repeat the word "relax" to yourself. "Relax. Relax. Relax."

Notice the feedback that you are getting from your body now compared to the way it felt before. It should be more relaxed, heavier, and perhaps you are feeling a tingling sensation throughout your body.

The final step of the Muscular Relaxation Response is to go back and concentrate on each body part you have already muscularly relaxed. You will concentrate on each part and tell it to relax five times. You will *not* contract your muscles at this time but simply concentrate and think of the repetition of the word "relax." This will allow you to remove any worrisome thoughts from your response system and facilitate the state of relaxation you have already achieved.

Think of your toes—Tell them to *RELAX, RELAX, RELAX, RELAX, RELAX.*

Think of your calves—Tell them to *RELAX, RELAX, RELAX, RELAX, RELAX.*

Think of your thighs—Tell them to *RELAX, RELAX, RELAX, RELAX, RELAX.*

Think of your buttocks—Tell them to *RELAX, RELAX, RELAX, RELAX, RELAX.*

Think of your stomach—Tell it to *RELAX, RELAX, RELAX, RELAX, RELAX.*

Think of your chest—Tell it to *RELAX, RELAX, RELAX, RELAX, RELAX.*

Think of your shoulders—Tell them to *RELAX, RELAX, RELAX, RELAX, RELAX.*

Think of your arms—Tell them to *RELAX, RELAX, RELAX, RELAX, RELAX.*

Think of your throat—Tell it to *RELAX, RELAX, RELAX, RELAX, RELAX.*

Think of the back of your neck and head—Tell them to *RELAX, RELAX, RELAX, RELAX, RELAX.*

Think of your face—Tell it to *RELAX, RELAX, RELAX, RELAX, RELAX.*

Appendix B

DEEP MUSCLE RELAXATION

Deep muscle relaxation is incompatible with anxiety. Muscle relaxation training consists of learning to tense and release various muscle groups throughout the body. An essential part of learning how to relax involves learning to pay close attention to the feelings of tension and relaxation in your body.

We employ tension in order to ultimately produce relaxation. Strong tension is noticeable, and you will learn to attend to these feelings. The initial production of tension gives us some momentum so that when we release the tension, deep relaxation is the result. Learning relaxation is like learning other motor skills. It will take some practice to become good at it.

Remove constraining items such as watches, rings, eyeglasses, contact lenses, and shoes, if desirable. Recline in a tilt-back chair or sit upright with feet firmly planted on the floor and arms lying loosely in your lap. Closing your eyes will often be helpful. Release tension immediately rather than gradually. Once a group of muscles is relaxed, do not move them unnecessarily.

Steps in Inducing Relaxation

1. Extend arms in front of you and clinch fists. For this and each successive muscle group, tense for 7 seconds and then rest muscles for 20-30 seconds before moving on to the next muscle group.

2. Extend arms in front of you and point fingers toward the ceiling as though you were pushing a wall.
3. Touch fingers to shoulders so as to tense biceps.
4. Shut eyes tightly so as to tense muscles around the eyes, in forehead, and temples (skip this exercise if you are wearing contact lens).
5. Push tongue against roof of mouth, clinch molar teeth, and pull corners of lips around as though trying to touch ears.
6. Pull chin down one inch from sternum (breast bone) and at the same time try to pull chin further toward sternum and backwards toward your back. This sets up antagonistic muscle reaction and causes head to tremor.
7. Take a deep breath and hunch shoulders up toward ears.
8. Pull shoulders back as though trying to touch them together in the back.
9. Suck stomach in as though trying to touch backbone.
10. Push rear end into chair so as to tense buttocks muscles.
11. Extend legs in front of you and lift heels six inches off floor so as to tense thigh muscles.
12. With legs extended and heels resting on floor, point toes toward knees so as to tense calf muscles.
13. With legs extended and heels resting on floor, curl toes under toward arches (tense for 3 seconds only as these muscles easily experience cramps).
14. Now, review the condition of each of these muscle groups and visualize them becoming more and more relaxed. See muscle fibers becoming looser and longer—stretching out like wet spaghetti. You may notice that your palms are becoming warmer, that your upper torso is becoming heavier and heavier. Concentrate on these effects since they are evidences of deep relaxation.

Sit quietly for several moments. You might wish to use this experience for implanting more firmly in your mind certain goals which are important to you. Picture the goal clearly in your mind, and see yourself reaching your goal. Make your picture as vivid and as much in detail as possible. You may find this is a great aid to your motivation.

Try to practice this exercise twice a day—morning and evening are best for most persons. Practice in the morning often helps in beginning the day more centered, less feverishly. Practice in the evening helps to wash out the cumulative stress of the day.

Used with permission of Regent's Professor and Director of Counseling Psychology Kenneth B. Matheny, Ph.D., Counseling and Psychological Services, Georgia State University, Atlanta, Georgia.

Appendix C

PRESCRIBED BREATHING

When we are relaxed or sleeping there is a natural rhythm to our breathing. The stomach slightly protrudes; the rib cage expands; and the shoulders lift slightly at the end of the cycle. This sequence of events occurs from the work of the diaphragmatic muscle. The diaphgram rests in a concave position during exhalation. During inhalation it contracts downward pulling the lungs which are attached to it down-and-outward, thus forming a vacuum.

When under stress, the natural rhythm of breathing is disturbed. We may hyperventilate by breathing rapidly and shallowly; or we may breathe too slowly and create hypoxia or hypoventilation. In either case the natural pH (hydrogen-ion concentration) level of the blood (normally 7.40) is disturbed. If the pH level increases sharply through hyperventilation, it causes *respiratory alkalosis* wherein oxygen is increased and carbon dioxide is decreased. If it moves sharply downward through hypoventilation, the result is *respiratory acidosis* wherein carbon dioxide is increased and oxygen decreased.

The effects of hyperventilation are quite common: dizziness, weakness and nervousness. Its effects can be lessened by having the person breathe in a paper sack since this will decrease oxygen and increase carbon dioxide. The person can achieve better results through balanced breathing. The formula for balanced or prescribed breathing was taken from an ancient Hindu yogic practice called Pranayama. Breathing in this prescribed manner will restore the natural pH condition and relieve the nervousness or anxiety.

Steps in Prescribed Breathing

1. Sit comfortably with feet firmly planted on the floor, body weight resting evenly on the spinal column, hands resting on lap, eyes closed, and garments appropriately loosened.
2. Before beginning the prescribed breathing, take your pulse. Count the beats for 30 seconds and double. After the breathing exercise, take your pulse once again. If you had an elevated pulse before beginning, the breathing exercise will often lower it a bit.
3. Inhale for 3 seconds; hold for 12 seconds; and exhale for 6 seconds.
4. On the sixth cycle hold your breath for 20 seconds and afterwards exhale explosively. Afterwards sit quietly for one minute while allowing your breathing to reach its own level.
5. Take your pulse for a second time while sitting quietly. If you were nervous to begin with, you will often show a lowered pulse.

Practice this exercise frequently until you can visualize the resulting relaxation before you begin. The more you practice it, the better the results. You might wish to use the experience to prepare yourself for those situations which are likely to make you anxious or angry. The entire experience takes roughly 2½ minutes.

Used with permission of Regent's Professor and Director of Counseling Psychology Kenneth B. Matheny, Ph.D., Counseling and Psychological Services, Georgia State University, Atlanta, Georgia.

Appendix D

GUIDELINES FOR PHYSICAL FITNESS

Scope of Fitness

To be physically fit one must have sufficient muscular strength, a safe margin of cardio-vascular endurance and an acceptable degree of flexibility of movement. All three aspects are important to fitness. While it is possible to be physically fit at the same time one has a serious health problem, usually fitness and health go together. Being fit has the added advantage of reducing the stressfulness of certain physical demands placed on us, of reducing fatigue and resulting emotional distress. The exercise regime necessary to maintain fitness is experienced by many as an excellent means of lowering stress.

Muscular Strength: You must first determine how much muscular strength you need for the activities that comprise your daily schedule. The body will normally develop the strength called for by these activities without any special effort on your part. You might like to pursue a modest weight training program, however, for one of two purposes: 1) to improve the cosmetic effect by the addition of muscle mass, and 2) to provide a margin of safety for those exceptional times when strenuous effort is required.

Flexibility: Flexibility is important both to the feeling of freedom within our bodies and to escape pulled muscles, tendons, and ligaments. The body tends to become less supple with age. Unless we specifically and systematically stretch the muscles and twist to the comfortable limits of our joints, we will find growing restrictions to physical movement. Perhaps the best single practice to fight this growing immobilization is *yoga*. Millions stay unbelievably agile through yoga. A splendid paperback ($2.75) offering step-by-step instruction through photographs is Richard Hittleman's *Yoga: 28 Day Exercise Plan*. N.Y.: Bantam Books, 1969. A second and simpler system, is suggested in *Feel Younger, Live Longer*, N.Y.: Rand McNally & Company, 1976.

Cardio-Vascular Endurance: Perhaps the most important aspect of physical fitness is the endurance capacity of the heart, lungs and blood vessels. While many factors have been implicated in the development of coronary artery disease, lack of adequate exercise appears to be a cardinal one. The heart and lungs are perfectly capable of improving their functioning enormously through aerobic exercise. Aerobic refers to exercise within one's breath, or exercise adjusted to the body's ability to supply adequate oxygen. There are many ways of exercising aerobically: jogging, cycling, swimming, skipping and aerobic dancing are excellent examples. The best exercises for the purpose of expanding the capacity of heart and lungs are those that call for sustained, rhythmic movements.

To be effective in improving coronary and pulmonary functioning the exercise should be performed steadily for a considerable amount of time, and persons should stay within their *training rates*. It is generally recommended that the exercise should last for 20–30 minutes. The training rate refers to the rate of the heart beat during the exercise. Actually we should speak of range rather than rate since it is acceptable to stay anywhere within a specified range of heart beats. The training range is computed by means of the following computation.

$$220 - \text{One's Age} \times \text{both } 70\% \text{ and } 85\%$$

This computation will result in two numbers. The smaller represents the lower limits of your training range, and the larger the upper. For example, if your age is 40, your training range is:

$$220 - 40 = 180 \times 70\% = 126 = \text{lower limit; and}$$
$$220 - 40 = 180 \times 85\% = 153 = \text{upper limit.}$$

You should exercise at a rate that will keep your heart rate between the lower and upper limits of your range. In the beginning you would do well to stay nearer the lower limit, but after your conditioning has improved considerable you can safely exercise toward the upper limit.

Exercising within the training range will produce the *training effect*. The training effect results in a strengthening of the heart, a slowing of the heart rate, improvement in the heart's efficiency, improved circulation, and improved transport of oxygen throughout the body. These highly desirable changes will contribute immensely to your energy level and reduce the likelihood of a heart attack from an unexpected increase in your work load. Furthermore, there is increasing evidence that aerobic exercise increases the concentration of High Density Lipoproteins (HDL) in the blood. HDL appears to significantly reduce the buildup of cholesterol along the lining of the vascular system and in this way lessens the likelihood of phlebitis, coronary infarction, and strokes. Jogging is presently the most popular of the aerobic exercises, and for this reason I am offering a few specific suggestions for your safety, profit and pleasure.

Jogging: If you choose to take up jogging, consider the following advice:

1. Check with your physician if you are middle aged or older, or if you have any reason for believing vigorous exercise might be contraindicated.
2. Purchase a good book to properly inform and inspire you as to the procedures and benefits of jogging. There are now many excellent volumes available. Two of the better are:

    Kenneth H. Cooper. *The New Aerobics.* N.Y.: Bantam Books, 1970. ($2.50).

    James F. Fixx. *The Complete Book of Running.* N.Y.: Random House Publishers, 1977.
3. Buy yourself some good equipment. Shoes are the most important item. Don't try to save money. Be prepared to spend $30.00 to $50.00. Wear as few clothes as you can and still be sufficiently warm and decent. Remember 40% of the body's energy goes into heat. After you have run for a few minutes, excess clothing will be unduly restrictive.
4. Plan to run-walk within your training range. If you are in poor condition, begin by walking briskly. Walk for three to five minutes, and

then check your pulse rate. If you suspect your rate exceeds 100, you will be able to monitor your rate by placing your hand over your heart. If below 100, you must take your pulse at the wrist or at the carotid artery in the neck. If you are unable to get your pulse within your training range by walking, run slowly for three minutes or so, and once again take your pulse. You can adequately estimate your pulse rate per minute by taking it for 6 seconds and adding a zero. This is equivalent to taking it for 60 seconds. If you have been run-ning, drop back to a walk while checking your pulse. Begin to take your pulse within three or four seconds after slowing to a walk since the heart beat will begin to slow after 10 seconds or so. If your pulse is within your training range, begin to slowly run again. Check your pulse every few minutes. If it begins to exceed your range, walk until it drops toward the lower limit, and then begin running again.

5. Jog for 20–30 minutes at each session. It is not necessary to jog each day; every other day will work fine.

6. Measure your running in minutes rather than miles. If you begin to compete against yourself in distance, you will push yourself harder than is desirable. You are likely to push past your training range in an effort to increase your mileage. If you are to run with others, explain that you must stay within your range, and invite them to run at your pace. Remember, "Gentle is the way." Running beyond your training range will not improve cardio-vascular endurance any faster than would be the case were you to remain within your range—and you might invite disaster.

7. Always warm up and cool down with various stretching exercises. Muscles in the back, upper and lower legs, and feet are particularly vulnerable to strain if not properly stretched before sustained running.

8. Make adjustments for extreme temperatures. Protect against frost-bite in bitter temperatures, and slow down considerably and drink plenty of liquids during severe heat and humidity.

9. Run erect with arms bent at the elbow and swinging freely forward and backward. Look 40–50 feet in front of you. Whenever possible, jog on grass, wood chips, or soft dirt areas. Always jog HEEL to TOE.

If you will heed these simple suggestions, you are likely to find the exercise extremely helpful in a rather short time. While you must exercise from three to six months to begin to get maximum benefit, significant benefits will be gotten in a few weeks.

GOOD LUCK. AND RUN IN GOOD HEALTH.

Used with permission of Regent's Professor and Director of Counseling Psychology Kenneth B. Matheny, Ph.D., Counseling and Psychological Services, Georgia State University, Atlanta, Georgia.

Appendix E

REFERENCES

Ahlem, A.H. *How to Cope with Conflict, Crisis, and Change.* Glendale, California: Regal Books, 1978.

Benet, G. *Patients and Their Doctors.* London: Balliere Tindale, 1979. .

Bryan, A.I. "Can there be a science of bibliotherapy?" *Library Journal,* 1939. 64: 773–776.

Cardenas, P.R. and Kutner, N.G. "The problem of fatigue in dialysis patients." *Nephron,* 1982. 30: 336–340.

Carter, L. *Good 'n' Angry.* Grand Rapids, Michigan: Baker Book House, 1983.

Chyatte, S.B. *On Borrowed Time: Living with Hemodialysis.* Oradell, New Jersey: Medical Economics, 1979.

Collins, G.R. *The Joy of Caring.* Waco, Texas: Word, Inc., 1980.

Cox-Gedmark, J. *Coping with Physical Disability.* Philadelphia: The Westminster Press, 1980.

Dyer, W. *Your Erroneous Zones.* New York: Funk & Wagnalls, 1976.

Fincher, P.F. "Bibliotherapy: rx-literature." *Southern Medical Journal,* 73, 2, 223–225.

Frankl, E.V. *Man's Search for Meaning.* Boston: Beacon Press, 1962.

Girdano, R. and Everly, E. *Controlling Stress and Tension: A Holistic Approach.* Englewood Cliffs, New Jersey: Prentice Hall, Inc., 1979.

Hadler, N.M. "Medical ramifications of the social security disability insurance program." *Annals of Internal Medicine,* 1982, 96, 665–669.

Harvey, A.M.; Johns, R.; Owens, A.; Ross, R. *The Principles and Practice of Medicine.* New York: Appleton–Century–Crofts, 1972.

Holvey, R. (ed.) *The Merck Manual.* Rohway, New Jersey: Merck and Co., Inc., 1972.

Jackson, E.N. *The Many Faces of Grief.* Nashville: The Parthenon Press, 1977.

Kaiser, R.B. "The way of the journal." *Psychology Today,* March, 1981, 64–72.

Kanfer, F.H. and Goldstien, A.P. *Helping People Change.* New York: Pergamon Press, 1980.

Krupp, N.E. "Adaptation to chronic illness." *Postgraduate Medicine,* November, 1976, 122-125.

Lanier, B.G. "The emotional and family aspects of dealing with lupus erythematosus." Speech given at Greater Atlanta Chapter, Lupus Foundation of America, Inc., April, 1981.

Lazarus, R.S. "Little hassles can be hazardous to your health." *Psychology Today,* July, 1981, 58–62.

Lewis, F.M. "Family level services for the cancer patient: critical distinctions, fallacies, and assessment." *Cancer Nursing.* June, 1983, 193-200.

Lindeman, E. "Symptomatology and management in acute grief." *Crisis intervention: Selected readings,* M.J. Parad (ed.), New York: Family Service Association of America, 1965.

Madden, M. *The Power to Bless.* Nashville: Broadman Press, 1970.

Marcel, G. *Homo Viator: Introduction to the Metaphysics of Hope.* New York: Harper Torch Books, 1962.

Melges, F.T. "Grief resolution therapy: reliving and revisiting." *American Journal of Psychotherapy,* January, 1980, 36, 51–61.

Money, J. "Sexual Problems in the Chronically Ill." *Sexual Problems, Diagnosis, and Treatment in Medical Practice.* C.W. Wahl (ed.). New York: Free Press, 1967.

Money, J. & Erhart, A. *Man and Woman, Boy and Girl.* New York: A Mentor Book, New American Library, 1972.

Moos, R.H. *Coping with Physical Illness.* New York: Plenum Medical Book Co., 1977.

NASA, "Warning: A weekend in bed can be hazardous to your health." *Family Circle,* March 29, 1983, 62.

Pearson, L. (ed.) *The Use of Written Communications in Psychotherapy*. Springfield, Illinois: Charles G. Thomas Publisher, 1965.

Powell, J. *Fully Human, Fully Alive*. Allen, Texas; Argus Communications, 1976. *Unconditional Love*. Allen, Texas: Argus Communications, 1978.

Progaff, I. *Process Meditation*. New York: Dialogue House, 1980.

Purtillo, R. "Similarities in patient response to chronic and terminal illness." *Physical Therapy*, 1976, 56, 279–284.

Raines, R. *To Kiss the Joy*. Waco, Texas: Word, Inc., 1977.

Rowat, K.M. The Meaning and Management of Chronic Pain: The Family's Perspective. Ann Arbor, Michigan: University Microfilms International, 1984, 3058.

Schrank, F.H. and Engels, P.W. "Bibliotherapy as a counseling adjunct: research findings." *The Personnel and Guidance Journal*, November, 1981, 143–147.

Shontz, C.S. *The Psychological Aspects of Physical Illness and Disability*. Reston, Virginia: Reston Publishing Co., Inc., 1975.

Wright, B.A. *Physical Disability: A Psychological Approach*. New York: Harper and Row, 1960.

Index